So you're having

Heart Bypass Surgery

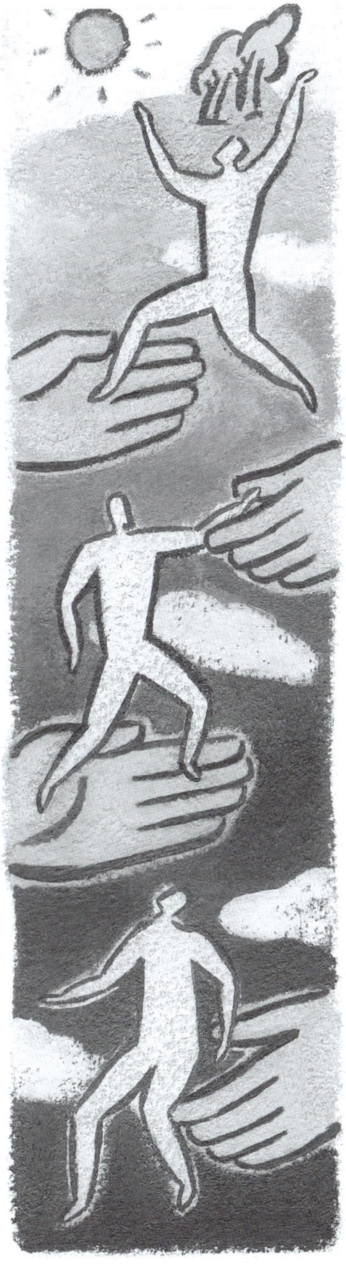

Tracey J. F. Colella RN
Suzette Turner RN
Bernard S. Goldman MD

PRESCRIPTION
℞ what happens next?™
SURGERY GUIDES

SCRIPT medical press inc.

First published in Canada in 2003 by
SCRIPT Medical Press, Inc.
Box 38096, 550 Eglinton Avenue West
Toronto, Ontario M5N 3A8
www.whathappensnext.ca

National Library of Canada Cataloguing in Publication
Colella, Tracey, 1967–
So you're having heart bypass surgery, what happens next?/
Tracey Colella, Suzette Turner, Bernard S. Goldman. — 1st
Canadian ed.

(What happens next ? surgery guides)
Includes bibliographical reference and index.
ISBN 0-9688982-1-1

1. Coronary artery bypass—Popular works. I. Goldman,
Bernard S., 1936– II. Turner, Suzette, 1966– III. Title.
IV. Series.

RD598.35.C67C64 2002 617.4'12 C2002-901497-2

Series Creator and General Editor: Helen Byrt
Editor: Jenny Lass
Copy editor: Andrea Knight
Book Design and Typesetting: Rocket Design
Cover Illustration: Ross Paul Lindo
Author Photographs: Al Gilbert, Doug Nicholson (Media Source)
Book Illustrations: Zane Waldman, Bernie Freedman

Publishing Consultant: Malcolm Lester & Associates

Printed and bound in Canada
03 04 05 54321

To all the patients and families
who are living this experience.
To my husband, Paul, my family,
Leslie, Judith, and Darryl,
and my close friend and colleague, Suzette;
they always inspire me.

T.J.F.C.

This book is dedicated to all my family and friends
who have been supportive
throughout this endeavor,
and to my patients.

S.T.

I dedicate this book to the thousands of patients
who have undergone CABG throughout my career,
and to the nurses and other health-care professionals
who contributed to their successful outcomes.

B.S.G.

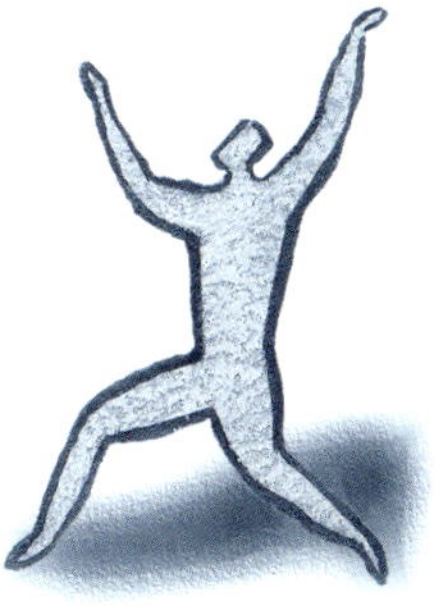

[FORTHCOMING BOOKS *in the* SERIES]

So You're Having
Prostate Surgery
—What Happens Next?

So You're Having A
Hysterectomy
—What Happens Next?

acknowledgments

Many fond thanks to Dr. Bernard Goldman for his mentoring, guidance, and ongoing support in this and all my pursuits. Thank you, with much gratitude, to the patients who have shared their personal insights and experiences with us. Thank you to Helen and the staff at SCRIPT for making this wonderful opportunity become a reality. Thank you to Dr. Stephen Fort for his greatly appreciated recommendation.

—Tracey J. F. Colella

I would like to thank Dr. Goldman for his guidance and support, Tracey, an inspiring friend, and our editor, whose support and vision have given this book life. Finally, a big thank you to our patients for providing us with the opportunity to be a part of your recovery.

—Suzette Turner

This book would not have been possible without the enthusiasm, creativity, expertise, and plain hard work of many individuals. We acknowledge with grateful thanks the financial support of Pfizer Canada Inc. Dr. Stephen Fort and Victoria Foulger RN generously gave us permission to use material from their own surgery guide, *So You're Having Angioplasty—What Happens Next*? Dr. Stuart McCluskey of the Physicians and Nurses for Blood Conservation tirelessly criticized the entire manuscript and injected his expertise into the sections on blood conservation and anesthetics. Harold Lass and Dr. Robert Maggisano cheerfully donated their services as models, for which we are grateful. Finally, many patients and families willingly shared their experiences of heart disease and bypass surgery with us: Arni Cohn, the late Robert (Bobby) Frew, Mrs. Joyce Frew, Dr. T. Hofmann, Cora Billing, Jim Morning, Ian Gillespie, Marie McVety, and Mel Isen. We thank you all.

—Helen Byrt

disclaimer

THE INFORMATION PROVIDED IN THIS BOOK MAY NOT apply to all patients, all clinical situations, all hospitals, or all eventualities, and is not intended to be a substitute for the advice of a qualified physician or other medical professional. Always consult a qualified physician about anything that affects your health, especially before starting an exercise program or using a complementary therapy not prescribed by your doctor.

The financial support received from the sponsors of this book does not constitute an endorsement by the authors or publisher of the sponsors or their products. Similarly, the naming of any organization, product or therapy in this book does not imply endorsement by the authors or publisher and the omission of any such names does not indicate disapproval by the authors or publisher.

contents

INTRODUCTION . . . xi

Chapter 1 — CORONARY ARTERY DISEASE AND YOU . . . 1
The facts on coronary artery disease ⁓ Reasons that you have clogged arteries ⁓ Symptoms ⁓ Taking control of your future

CHAPTER 2 — DIAGNOSING YOUR HEART DISEASE . . . 10
Overview of coronary angiography ⁓ Understanding your angiogram—and your diagnosis

CHAPTER 3 — IS BYPASS SURGERY RIGHT FOR YOU? . . . 15
Reasons for recommending bypass ⁓ Your other options ⁓ Pros and cons of bypass surgery, angioplasty, and medication alone

CHAPTER 4 — GETTING READY FOR YOUR BYPASS SURGERY . . . 29
Meeting your surgeon ⁓ Questions you could ask ⁓ Consent ⁓ Blood-transfusion options ⁓ Pre-surgery tests and arrangements

CHAPTER 5 — THE DAY OF YOUR BYPASS SURGERY . . . 41
Your hospital checklist ⁓ Arrival at the hospital ⁓ Preparations for surgery

CHAPTER 6 — THE CORONARY BYPASS PROCEDURE . . . 47
Step-by-step guide to the procedure ⁓ General anesthetic ⁓ Bypass grafts ⁓ Heart-lung machine ⁓ Closing the incision

CHAPTER 7 — NON-TRADITIONAL BYPASS SURGERY 65
Pros and cons of non-traditional approaches ~ Step-by-step guide to beating-heart surgery ~ Other minimally invasive surgery

CHAPTER 8 — WHEN IT'S ALL OVER 71
What to expect when you wake up ~ Intensive care unit ~ Your recovery in the ward ~ Managing pain ~ Getting mobile ~ Wound care ~ Treating complications ~ Leaving hospital

CHAPTER 9 — RECOVERING AT HOME 85
When and where to get help ~ Sleeping, driving, eating, sex ~ Getting back on your feet ~ Cardiac rehabilitation ~ Back to work ~ Caring for your incision ~ Medications ~ Dealing with pain ~ Dealing with the blues

CHAPTER 10 — HOW YOU CAN HELP YOURSELF 99
Take control and transform your future ~ Diet ~ Exercise ~ Learn to relax ~ Complementary therapies

CHAPTER 11 — HAS MY BYPASS SURGERY WORKED? 118
How you might feel right away ~ What to expect over the next year ~ The long-term picture

CHAPTER 12 — MEDICATIONS 124
Making the most of your meds ~ Treatments for heart disease ~ Medications before, during and after surgery

CHAPTER 13 — FUTURE DIRECTIONS IN CARDIAC SURGERY . . 135
Taking part in a clinical trial ~ Up-coming technologies

CHAPTER 14 — WHO'S WHO OF HOSPITAL STAFF 139

GLOSSARY 145
RESOURCES 152
YOUR DIARY 156
INDEX 162

introduction

The purpose of this book is to introduce you and your family to coronary bypass graft surgery. Although bypass surgery is the most common major operation performed in the world, with 600,000 procedures conducted each year in North America alone, the decision to undergo heart surgery may be difficult. Our goal is to familiarize you with the concepts and controversies regarding this remarkable procedure so that you can make a fully informed decision about your operation.

Before the 1960s there were no operations to directly improve blood flow to the heart muscle. Although surgeons had tried many ingenious procedures, none was very successful in relieving angina. It was not until 1962, when coronary angiography was first performed, that cardiologists could get a direct look at blockages in the blood vessels of the heart and provide cardiac surgeons with a "road map" to bypass the obstructions. The first coronary bypass was reported in 1967, and the procedure was rapidly and enthusiastically taken up by surgeons. However, the operation was soon criticized by some doctors who felt that better use of medicines, rather than surgery, was still the answer. There were also concerns about how to choose the patients most likely to benefit, the risks involved, and the early setbacks that occurred when only vein grafts were used. Luckily, important clinical studies carried out in the 1970s in North America and Europe soon confirmed the low risk and incredible benefit of the operation.

Coronary bypass graft surgery has evolved and matured over the years and remains the gold standard for many patients, especially those with many blocked arteries, poor heart-muscle contraction, and significant narrowing in the important left main coronary artery. Because similar advances have been made in the other treatments for angina—medications and angioplasty (introduced in 1977)— patients can now benefit from a combined approach to their coronary disease. And improvements will continue. New operating-room techniques and improved recovery programs, with a greater emphasis on reducing risks through medication and lifestyle changes, should further brighten the outlook for people with heart disease.

It has been said that more scientific papers have been written about coronary bypass graft surgery than any other operation in medical history. While this is difficult to prove, it is certainly true that bypass graft surgery has been intensely studied over three decades and has shown to be safe and effective in the majority of people. Our hope is that your bypass surgery will change your life for the better.

Good luck!

Chapter 1

coronary artery disease and you

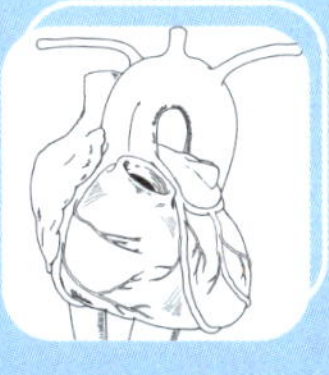

What Happens in this Chapter

- The facts on coronary artery disease
- The likely reasons you have clogged arteries
- The symptoms of angina and a heart attack
- How you can take control of your future

Your heart is a pump the size of your fist. It beats about 60 times a minute to keep blood circulating through your body, carrying nutrients and oxygen to your tissues. It is made of a unique type of muscle called ***myocardium****—the only muscle in the body that keeps contracting without needing a break. The blood supply that allows the myocardium to do this comes from the coronary arteries. When the coronary arteries get blocked by disease, the blood supply to the myocardium is interrupted, resulting in angina or a heart attack. The aim of surgery is to bypass the blockage and restore normal blood flow to the myocardium.*

How the Heart Works

The human heart is an amazing piece of engineering. It is actually two pumps in one: the right half of the heart pumps blood to the lungs to pick up oxygen, while the left half receives the oxygen-rich blood from the lungs and pumps it onwards, around the rest of the body. Valves inside the heart keep the blood moving in the right direction and a thin, lubricated membrane outside (called the **pericardium**) ensures that the pumping heart can move easily.

The heart muscle itself (the myocardium) needs a good blood supply to keep contracting, especially during exercise or exertion. The arteries that supply the heart muscle with blood are called the **coronary arteries**—so-called because from above they look like a crown. The coronary arteries branch off the **aorta** (the main blood vessel in your body) at the point where the oxygen-rich blood leaves the heart and course over the surface of the heart. The heart is the first organ in your body to receive oxygenated blood, and is unique in that it must supply its own nutrition.

Coronary Artery Disease

Coronary artery disease is a condition in which one or more of the coronary arteries becomes narrowed, so that the heart muscle does not receive enough oxygen. Both angina and heart attacks are usually caused by coronary artery disease, which is the leading cause of death and disability in developed countries.

Coronary artery disease is a form of **atherosclerosis**—a process where the arteries gradually clog up like old water pipes. Over several decades, cholesterol, calcium, and other substances build up on and under the artery's inner lining, creating a narrowing that starts to block the flow of blood down the artery (see Figure 1–1). The technical term for this blockage is a **plaque.**

Figure 1–1. How a Plaque Develops

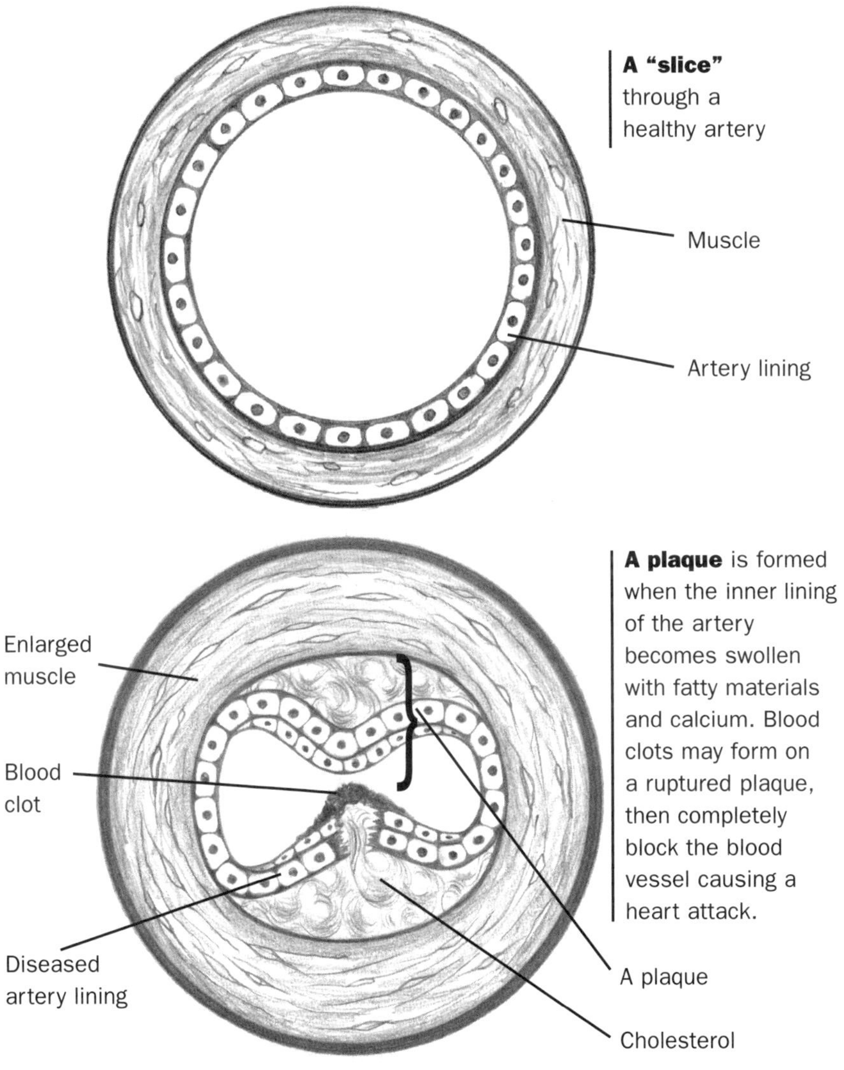

> "When I was first in the hospital and we thought it was a heart attack, I was upset. My wife said, 'Settle down. It's not the end of the world.' And I did sort of sit back and say, 'Well, at least I'm still alive.'"
>
> **Jim Morning**

Plaques can become surprisingly large before they start to restrict blood flow because, at first, the artery does its best to compensate for the blockage by stretching and expanding its outer wall. However, this so-called "positive remodeling" has its limits, and gradually the inside of the artery becomes so narrowed that blood flow is reduced, and the symptoms of angina start to appear.

Why Do You Have Coronary Artery Disease?

It is still not clear what triggers coronary artery disease, despite many years of research. It can start as early as the teenage years: post-mortem studies on young soldiers who died during the Vietnam War showed that they had early signs of atherosclerosis. It is clear, however, that there are a number of factors that increase people's chances of getting coronary artery disease—so-called **cardiac risk factors.** These include lifestyle choices such as smoking and lack of exercise, as well as "unmodifiable" risk factors, such as a family history of heart disease (see Key Point box).

The good news is that if you change the risk factors in your life you can improve your future health considerably, even if you already have coronary artery disease.

KEY POINT

Major risk factors for coronary artery disease

Nothing is certain in life, but if you have one or more of these risk factors, then you are more likely to develop coronary artery disease. The more severe the risk factor, the more severe your coronary artery disease is likely to be.

- Family history
- Hyperlipidemia (e.g., high blood cholesterol)
- Smoking
- Diabetes
- High blood pressure
- Obesity
- Sedentary lifestyle

Angina

Usually, the first sign of coronary artery disease is **angina**, a chest pain that starts during exercise and gets better during rest. Most commonly, angina feels like a dull, heavy, constricting sensation that starts in the center of the chest and may spread into the throat or down one arm. However, it varies greatly from person to person and may feel like jaw or back pain.

Angina happens when there is an inadequate supply of blood to the myocardium. The heart muscle becomes starved of oxygen and toxins build up, causing cramp-like pain. It is also called **myocardial ischemia**—literally, a reduction of blood to the heart muscle. Angina usually appears first during physical exercise or emotional stress because the heart is beating faster and more strongly, and thus requires more oxygen.

Figure 1–2. The Coronary Arteries

These small but crucial arteries supply blood (and oxygen) to the muscle of the heart itself. There are three main arteries—the **right coronary artery** and the two branches of the left coronary artery (the **left anterior descending artery** and the **circumflex artery**).

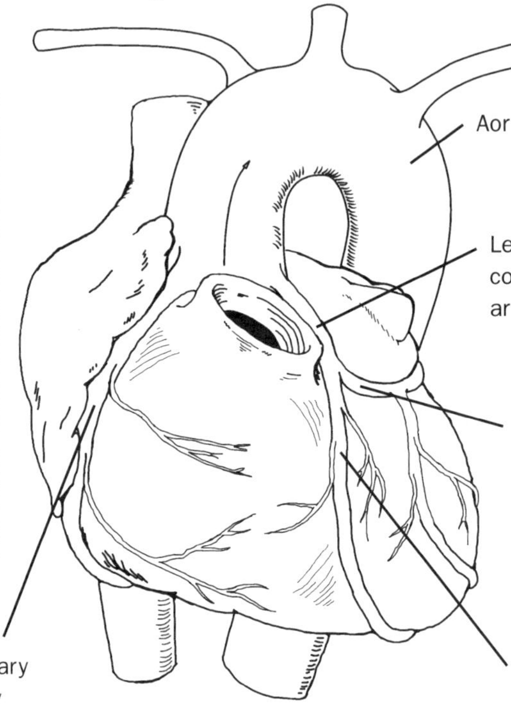

If the blockages in the coronary arteries become severe, angina may be experienced even when resting. This is called **unstable angina**, and is a serious condition: a small number of patients who develop this form of severe angina are likely to have a heart attack within the next few weeks or months.

Not everyone feels pain with angina. "Painless" angina (also known as **silent ischemia**) can show up on an electrocardiogram (ECG), although the patient may be unaware of it or experience it as a non-painful symptom such as breathlessness. Silent ischemia is more common than was previously thought, and it may be due to shorter, or less severe, episodes of ischemia than those causing typical angina symptoms. Silent ischemia is treated in the same way as typical angina.

Although angina is most commonly caused by coronary artery disease, it can occasionally result from other heart conditions, for instance a disease of the heart valve called **aortic stenosis.**

A Heart Attack

> "Back in 1965 we didn't even know there was such a thing as angina. I think my Mum had it, but they all thought 'pleurisy'—nobody spoke about angina. Father had a coronary thrombosis, too, so it does run in the family."
>
> **Robert (Bobby) Frew**

In angina, blood still flows down the coronary artery and some oxygen reaches the heart muscle. By contrast, in a heart attack (or **myocardial infarction**), the coronary artery is blocked very suddenly and completely, causing a small area of muscle to die and a scar to form. The symptoms of a heart attack are usually different from the symptoms of angina (see Key Point box on page 8).

Many heart attacks occur in people with no previous warning signs of angina. In addition, up to one quarter of heart attacks are "silent," without any chest pain. The cause of such silent heart attacks is currently unknown. However, since they are more common in people with diabetes—who often have damaged nerves—one theory is that silent heart attacks may result from abnormalities in the nerves that supply the heart, so people simply don't feel the pain.

Every chest pain is not angina or a heart attack. There can be many other reasons for chest pain, for instance, indigestion or pneumonia. Always see your physician if you experience pains in your chest.

> "When I had my heart attack it was the first indication of any heart problem. I had some shortness of breath, but never made the connection."
>
> **Arni Cohn**

If you have coronary artery disease, it is likely that you also have atherosclerosis in other arteries of your body. This means that you are at greater risk of having a stroke (due to atherosclerosis in the blood vessels of the brain) or poor circulation in other vital organs such as your kidneys. But don't despair. The future is in your hands. Remember, only one cardiac risk factor can't be altered—your family history. Everything else can be changed and it is never too early or too late to start. For advice on what you can do to help yourself, see Chapter 10.

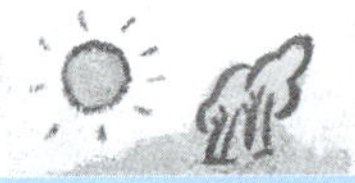

KEY POINT

If you have the following symptoms you are more likely to be having a heart attack than angina

- Severe, heavy, crushing pain in your chest
- Pain that lasts more than 20 to 30 minutes
- Pain that does not go away when you rest
- No relief from sublingual nitroglycerine
- Breathlessness
- Nausea and, sometimes, vomiting
- Fainting or lightheadedness
- Rapid heartbeat
- Pallor and sweating

If you think you are having a heart attack, dial 911 right away. Do not waste time calling your cardiologist or family doctor.

What Happens Next?

If your physician thinks you have angina, there are a number of ways to confirm that you have it, find out the reason for it, and decide how serious it is. You may be sent for "non-invasive" tests such as an exercise stress test, or **treadmill test**, a **nuclear perfusion scan**, or an **echocardiogram** (see Glossary for details of these tests), which will show how well your heart is working. You may then be sent for **coronary angiography**, an "invasive" test that involves placing a tube (catheter) into your body to see what state your coronary arteries are in. Coronary angiography is covered in the next chapter. Your physician may also prescribe lipid-lowering medication at this stage to slow down the progression of atherosclerosis throughout your body, ASA (Aspirin) to reduce the risk of having a heart attack by thinning the blood, and anti-anginal drugs to relieve your angina symptoms.

"One of the things people have to understand, and this is something I got afterwards, is that we have heart disease. This is a disease. It's not going to go away—but it can be controlled."

Mel Isen

Chapter 2

diagnosing your heart disease

What Happens in this Chapter

- Overview of coronary angiography
- Understanding your angiogram—and your diagnosis

Coronary angiography gives you and your medical team the inside story on your heart. It is not a treatment, but a diagnostic tool—a way of finding out exactly what is wrong with you. By injecting a special dye into the arteries of your heart and looking at the X-ray picture on a TV screen in real time, your physician can see which blood vessels are blocked, where, and how badly. This will help him or her to decide whether you need bypass surgery, angioplasty, or just drug therapy.

What is Coronary Angiography?

An angiogram is an X-ray picture of your heart's own blood supply, and the most useful information that you and your medical team could have. Most people reading this book will have already had an angiogram, so the procedure itself is only covered briefly here. For a step-by-step guide to having an angiogram, see the book *So You're Having Angioplasty—What Happens Next?* (see page 153).

There are three main coronary arteries that supply blood to the heart muscle (see page 6). During your angiogram your physician will check all three arteries for disease. Blood vessels don't normally

Figure 2–1. Cardiac Catheterization

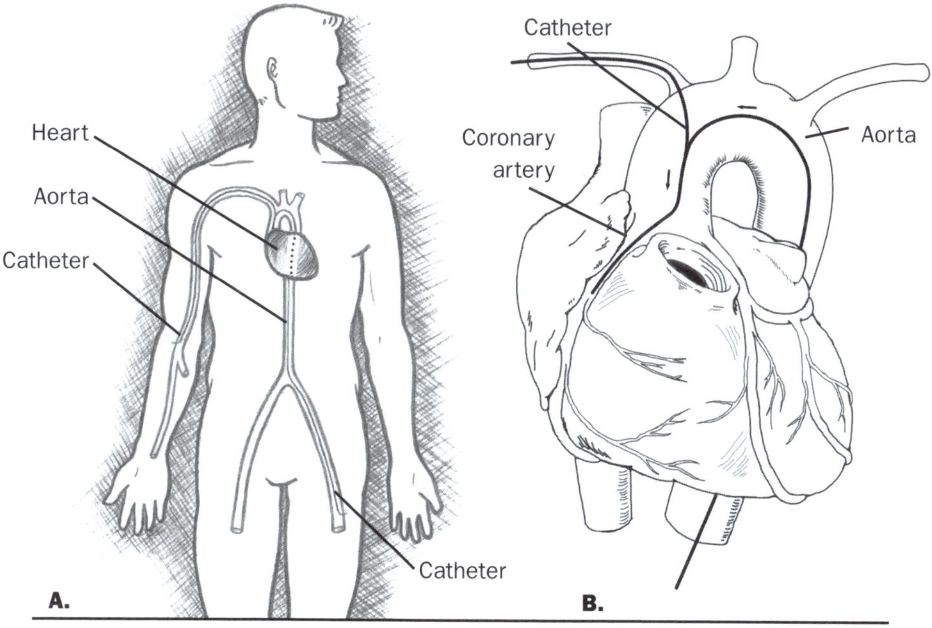

Angiography and angioplasty use this technique, in which a tube called a catheter is inserted into the heart's blood vessels via an artery in the arm or the groin (A). The catheter is then used to inject radio-opaque dye and insert angioplasty equipment into the coronary arteries (B).

[MORE DETAIL]

Single-, double-, or triple-vessel disease — Disease in one, two, or three of the coronary arteries (for more on coronary arteries, see Figure 1–2, page 6).

A plaque — The technical term for the blockage in your coronary artery. Plaques are made of cholesterol, scar tissue, and, sometimes, calcium.

Stenosis — A narrowing in a coronary artery, caused by a plaque; classified as mild, moderate, or severe, or expressed as a percentage. An artery can become 70 percent narrowed before symptoms of angina appear. Blockages of 20 to 50 percent are a sign of early disease, do not necessarily result in angina, and are usually treated with medication and diet.

Left main disease — Disease in the left (main) coronary artery, the most important blood vessel of the heart. If this vessel is severely diseased, bypass surgery is usually recommended, although angioplasty may be possible.

Occlusion — A total blockage (100 percent) of the vessel. Chronic occlusions (a blockage over 6 months old) can be very difficult to unblock by angioplasty. Even if successful, the re-narrowing rate after angioplasty is high. Bypass surgery is usually preferred in this situation.

Impaired left ventricular function — The pumping action of the main chamber of the heart (the left ventricle). This is often impaired after a heart attack, in which case bypass surgery is more likely to be recommended.

show up on X-rays, so an angiogram is created by injecting a dye that is visible to X-rays into the blood vessels of the heart. This is done by passing a fine tube into an artery in the groin or arm and pushing it all the way along to the heart—a procedure called **cardiac catheterization** (see Figure 2–1).

Angiography is the "gold standard" diagnostic test for coronary artery disease, but other techniques are being developed and may become more common in the future. **Electron beam computer tomography** (EBCT) uses large doses of radiation to measure the calcium in coronary arteries. **Magnetic resonance imaging** (MRI) is also being explored for coronary artery disease, although it is currently not as accurate (or as useful) as angiography.

Figure 2–2. Coronary Angiogram

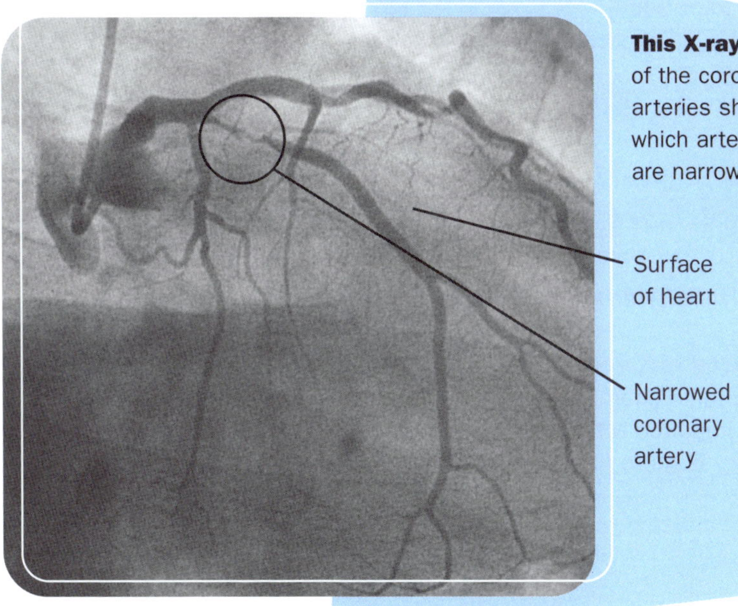

This X-ray picture of the coronary arteries shows which arteries are narrowed.

Diagnosing Your Heart Disease

After your angiogram your physician should be able to tell you exactly what is wrong, how serious your heart disease is, and what treatment will be best for you.

In general, mild disease (less than 50 percent narrowing) of one, two, or three coronary arteries is usually treated with medication and diet. In moderate disease, where 50 to 70 percent of the artery is blocked, treatment depends on how bad your symptoms are and the results of other cardiac tests. Severe "single-vessel" disease (more than 70 percent narrowing of one artery) is usually treated with angioplasty. Severe "three-vessel" disease is more likely to be treated with coronary artery bypass surgery.

What Happens Next?

In most people, angiography gives clear answers and the next steps are obvious. If not, you may need to attend one or more further clinic appointments for some extra tests. If your physician recommends bypass surgery or angioplasty, you will be referred to a specialist as the next step. The next chapter explains more about your treatment choices.

Chapter 3

is bypass surgery right for you?

What Happens in this Chapter

- How your health-care team decides which treatment to recommend
- People who benefit most from bypass surgery
- Your treatment options
- Pros and cons of bypass surgery, angioplasty, and medication alone

If you have heart disease, you do not necessarily have to have bypass surgery. Angioplasty or drug treatment alone may be the best option for you. Even if your medical team strongly recommends bypass surgery based on your own medical situation, it is worth knowing about the alternatives —and the pros and cons of bypass surgery— so that you are fully informed before giving your consent for the procedure.

The Treatment Decision

Once your coronary angiogram and other tests have confirmed that you have heart disease, you and your physician will need to agree on the best treatment.

Any decision about a medical treatment involves balancing risks and benefits. The goal of your treatment should be to relieve any chest discomfort, increase your level of activity, improve your quality of life, and prolong your life—with the least possible risk.

Heart disease can be treated with either drug therapy, angioplasty, or coronary artery bypass surgery. Your physician will make recommendations based on his or her past experience with patients whose medical situation is similar to yours, other medical conditions you may have, and his or her knowledge of the most recent scientific studies.

The choice may be obvious. For instance, you may have had a heart attack due to a blockage that can be easily opened with angioplasty. Or, you may have significant disease in the crucial left main coronary artery, in which case a bypass is needed. When the decision is less clear-cut, practical considerations—such as how quickly you need to return to work—can play a part.

"I was very surprised. I thought that in the worst case they might say, 'You better cut back on your saturated fats and exercise a bit more.' I did not anticipate heart surgery."

Ian Gillespie

This chapter summarizes the advantages and disadvantages of drug therapy alone, bypass surgery, and angioplasty, based on the most recently available scientific information and the experience of the authors. Our intention is to give you enough information to be able to make an informed decision about your treatment.

[SELF-HELP]

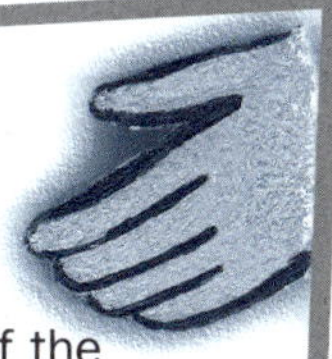

How to Decide?

- Your own health situation may mean that one or more of the options in this chapter are not available to you. However, it's still worth knowing the advantages and disadvantages of your own treatment so that you are fully informed before you sign the consent form.

- If in doubt, a second opinion from another physician can sometimes help.

- As with all illnesses, your heart disease can change over time and you may need to revise your decision.

- You are entitled to change your mind if you feel that you have made the wrong choice.

- For more information on angioplasty, see the book, *So You're Having Angioplasty—What Happens Next?* (page 152).

If you and your physician have already decided that bypass surgery is the best choice for you, this chapter will give you the information that you need before signing your consent form.

Drug Treatment

All patients with heart disease are treated with medication, whether or not they have surgery. You may be taking several different drugs—

some to relieve your angina, others to reduce the risks of a heart attack, and still others aimed at slowing the progression of your disease. (For a detailed discussion of medications, see Chapter 12.)

With the large number of potent and effective drugs currently available, many patients with mild or moderate heart disease can be successfully treated by drug therapy alone. Obviously, the main advantage of this is that you don't have to undergo the discomfort, inconvenience, or risks of a hospital procedure.

The disadvantage of drug treatment alone is the sheer number of medications you will have to take—and their cost. By contrast, after successful angioplasty or bypass surgery you *may* be able to cut down on the number of drugs you take because you will no longer need to take medication for your angina symptoms. However, you will need to continue taking medicine for other conditions such as high blood pressure.

The more drugs you take and the higher their doses, the more likely you are to suffer drug side effects. A list of the common side effects associated with heart medications is given in Chapter 12. It is impossible for your physician to predict whether you will suffer any side effects. Bear in mind, too, that it is impossible for him or her to give any guarantees about how well your angina will respond to medication, or which drug will be most effective. A period of trial and error is often needed before your physician can find the right combination of drugs—and doses—to suit you.

Despite these limitations, drug therapy may be the right long-term option for you if you are unhappy about the risks of a hospital procedure and if your angina is well controlled—that is, if your angina attacks are infrequent and you can lead a normal or near-normal life with few or no restrictions.

Remember, if your angina gets worse in the future, you can always change your mind and ask your physician to refer you for angioplasty or bypass surgery.

What is Bypass Surgery?

Coronary artery bypass surgery was first reported in 1967 and has since undergone many improvements. A heart surgeon creates a "bypass" around the blocked or narrowed coronary artery by using a blood vessel taken from elsewhere in your body. The resulting bypass is called a **coronary artery bypass graft** or **CABG** (pronounced "cabbage"). Thus, bypass surgery does not itself attempt to unblock the coronary arteries—it simply creates another route for the blood to reach the heart muscle. For a step-by-step description of the procedure, see Chapters 6 and 7.

What Is Angioplasty?

Angioplasty involves unblocking your narrowed coronary arteries by inserting a small balloon into each artery and inflating the balloon at the site of the narrowing. This presses the blockage to the sides of the artery and stretches the artery slightly, allowing blood to flow freely once more. A small tube called a **stent** is usually inserted at the same time to hold the artery open. Angioplasty involves making a small puncture in either the arm or the groin to insert the balloon equipment all the way up to the heart. The experience is similar to angiography—the procedure that was used to diagnose your heart disease. For more on angioplasty see the book, *So You're Having Angioplasty—What Happens Next?* (details on page 152).

[KEY POINT]

If your angina is NOT well controlled by your medication, for example, if you experience angina when doing nothing to provoke an attack, or you suffer recurrent or prolonged episodes of angina, you should tell your doctor immediately.

Bypass Surgery

Increased Life Expectancy

A major advantage of bypass surgery is that it appears to be more effective in prolonging life and prevent heart attacks *in some people*, compared to angioplasty or just taking medicines. Sicker patients appear to benefit most (see More Detail box on page 22). These include people with severe disease of the left main artery, disease in all three arteries *and* a weakened heart pumping action, or diabetic people with disease in two or more vessels.

However, even if you have these conditions, don't be surprised if your physician still offers you the choice of angioplasty. There are no hard and fast rules in choosing one treatment over another, especially as angioplasty and stents have advanced greatly in recent years and may now be as effective as bypass surgery for some of these sicker patients.

Angioplasty or medicines alone will probably be as effective as bypass surgery if you have stable heart disease, no other medical conditions such as diabetes, a good heart pumping action, and only one or two blockages. As always, your physician will advise you, based on your own health.

Good Angina Control

Bypass surgery is a very effective treatment for angina. Within the first year, only about 3 percent of people experience a return of their angina symptoms, compared to 10 to 20 percent for angioplasty and stent insertion (or 20 to 30 percent for angioplasty alone).

Improved Quality of Life

Most people find that their quality of life is much better following bypass surgery than it was before surgery. Within 6 weeks many feel

Survival Rates after Bypass Surgery

[MORE DETAIL]

You will read many different survival rates for bypass surgery. Survival varies widely depending on age, type of heart disease, and whether you have had a recent heart attack or other medical problems. The survival rates below are averages for younger patients (i.e., under 60 years of age) with stable heart disease. However, bear in mind that these figures are for surgery performed in the 1970s and 1980s, involving vein grafts only. Medical improvements since then—especially the use of artery grafts—mean even better survival for today's patients.

Number of Years	**Survival**	
	Bypass Surgery	Medicines Only
1	95%	95%
5	90%	84%
7	84%	78%
10	74%	69%

well enough to return to work and after 3 months, most patients can resume a normal, physically active life. (For more on recovery timelines, see page 121).

Benefits Sicker Patients and Patients with Diabetes

A major advantage of bypass surgery is that it can treat patients that angioplasty cannot. Because it can bypass the entire coronary artery, bypass surgery is useful for patients with multiple blockages in one or more arteries. By providing a new route, it can also deal with

> "Get it done. It's no big deal anymore."
>
> **Jim Morning**

long-term, hard blockages that are impossible to open with angioplasty, or with stents that have become blocked after angioplasty. Also, as discussed earlier, bypass surgery *may* give better long-term prospects than angioplasty for sicker patients, such as patients with disease in the critical left main artery, or diabetic patients with two or more blockages.

All Surgery Will Be Over at Once

Bypass surgery is the obvious option for your angina if you also need another heart procedure, for instance valve surgery, that requires opening up your chest. This way you get everything done at once, and you won't have to come back into the hospital for bypass surgery later if your coronary heart disease gets worse.

[MORE DETAIL]

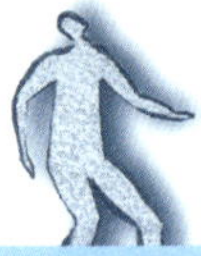

You may benefit more from bypass surgery than angioplasty if you have:

- had a failed angioplasty or your stent has become blocked
- a coronary artery that has been completely blocked for several weeks or months
- damaged heart valves or other condition that requires heart surgery
- coronary arteries narrowed in more than one place
- blockages in all three coronary arteries AND a weakened left ventricle
- diabetes AND more than one blocked artery
- severe narrowing in the left main coronary artery

The Downsides of Bypass Surgery

A Major Procedure

Although bypass surgery is one of the most widely performed surgeries in the Western world, it is still major surgery. It takes at least four hours to perform, involves opening up your chest, requires a general anesthetic, and, in most cases, a heart-lung machine. You may take weeks or months to recover. By contrast, angioplasty takes one hour or less, and recovery is faster—days or weeks only.

Grafts

Bypass surgery involves grafting a vein or artery from elsewhere in the body onto the heart to bypass the blocked artery. The grafts can be taken from leg veins, or arteries in the arm or chest. This means that you will have additional discomfort in your arm or leg as the scars heal. Angioplasty does not involve any surgical incisions.

Visible Scars

Obviously, with bypass surgery there is an incision in the chest, and—for the blood vessels used as grafts—leg or arm incisions. The scars will take time to heal and may become infected.

The Heart-Lung Machine

The **heart-lung** or **cardiopulmonary bypass (CPB) machine** revolutionized heart surgery in the late 1960s by allowing surgeons to work on a heart that was not beating by taking over the job of pumping blood around the body. This meant that

> "I was 64 years old and I wasn't able to do a whole lot...I thought that if I could get this thing over with and get better, why not?"
>
> **Jim Morning**

surgeons could help more patients than ever before. However, there are downsides to the heart-lung machine, such as an increased risk of fluid retention, kidney impairment, or needing a blood transfusion. The heart-lung machine may also be at least partly responsible for the short-term memory and concentration problems experienced by some patients after bypass surgery (see page 26).

Be assured that, if you do need the heart-lung machine, your health-care team will be working hard to minimize any long-term problems. Some surgeons are now performing **beating-heart surgery** to avoid the heart-lung machine altogether, although this technique has its own risks (see Chapter 7).

Greater Risk of Blood Transfusion

Blood transfusion is more likely with bypass surgery than with angioplasty—at least 10 percent of bypass patients require a blood transfusion. By contrast, a blood transfusion is rarely needed after angioplasty. Beating-heart surgery, in which the heart-lung machine is not used (Chapter 7), slightly reduces the chances of a blood transfusion compared to traditional bypass surgery.

Other Risks

Like all medical procedures, bypass surgery has other risks. For the last 40 years, surgeons have been studying what makes one person recover well from bypass surgery while another has problems. We now know that—not surprisingly—a person's general health at time of surgery is the most important factor that determines how well they will recover from the procedure. In general, older and sicker

Major Risks of Bypass Surgery

[MORE DETAIL]

- Death in "low-risk" patients (1 to 3 percent)
- Heart attack (3 to 5 percent)
- Stroke (1 to 5 percent)
- Concentration and memory problems (estimates vary widely, from insignificant to one-quarter of patients at 6 months)
- Blood transfusion (10 percent or more)
- Return of angina (3 percent in first year)

See also page 81 for problems you may encounter in the hospital.

Major Risks of Angioplasty

- Death (less than 0.1 percent)
- Heart attack (2 to 5 percent)
- Stroke (0.5 percent)
- Sudden blockage of coronary artery, resulting in emergency bypass surgery (less than 1 percent)
- Blood transfusion (0.5 percent)
- Return of angina (10 to 20 percent with stent)

patients encounter more problems than younger, healthier patients—although this is a generalization and may not apply in your case. Your physician will weigh the benefit of bypass surgery against the possible risks to you. Everyone's case is different, so always be guided by your physician.

Stroke

A stroke happens when a part of the brain becomes starved of oxygen, either because of a blockage in the blood flow to the brain

Angioplasty may be a better option for you than bypass surgery if you have

[MORE DETAIL]

- had a very recent heart attack
- severe lung disease (e.g., emphysema)
- any medical condition that means you shouldn't have a general anesthetic
- had a past stroke
- serious kidney disease
- diseased arteries elsewhere in the body (circulation problems)
- had one or more bypass operations already

tissue or internal bleeding in the brain. The symptoms of stroke vary widely, depending on which part of the brain is affected, from unconsciousness to weakness in an arm or leg. Strokes are a possibility after any surgery. Strokes after bypass surgery happen in 1 to 5 percent of people. They are more likely in the elderly and people who have had a stroke before. They are also more common in people with an existing blockage in the blood vessels of the neck and head, so your health-care team will check you carefully before surgery. If they find a blockage, your physician may recommend that the blockage be cleared before bypass surgery, using a procedure called **carotid endarterectomy**.

Cognitive deficits

For reasons that are still not clear, cognitive deficits—changes in memory, concentration, and reaction times—are relatively common after bypass surgery. They happen more often in older patients, patients with heart failure, and patients who have had a heart attack. They are also more common after longer, more complicated operations. Some of the cognitive defects may be related to fatigue, anemia, or painkillers, as in any operation. The heart-lung machine is also thought to cause microscopic brain changes that take time to heal. The effects are worse immediately after surgery (about 50 percent of patients are affected at hospital discharge) and get better over time (about 24 percent of patients at 6 months). Within a year, most people recover to a point at which their normal lives are not affected, although some may complain of feeling "not right" for longer than this.

Risk of death

The risk of dying during or shortly after bypass surgery is around 2 percent. This is an average, and your own personal risk may be much lower than this, depending on many factors—most importantly, your health status before surgery. Your physician will carefully consider your own particular risks before recommending bypass surgery.

What Happens Next?

There are many factors to consider when contemplating heart bypass surgery. If you are unsure about what your physician is recommending, it may be worth seeking a second opinion from another physician. Don't feel embarrassed to do this because, at the end of the day, you are the one having surgery, not your doctor.

It is worth remembering, too, that although bypass surgery can relieve your angina, it does not actually cure your heart disease. Even if you have bypass surgery, you still need to make changes that will improve the health of your heart, otherwise your heart disease will continue to get worse. Take your medication correctly and don't forget to make lifestyle changes (see Chapter 10). Heart disease is a wake-up call: it's time to choose a different road.

Chapter 4

getting ready for your heart bypass surgery

What Happens in this Chapter

- Meeting with your cardiac surgeon
- Common questions before surgery
- Consent
- Blood transfusions and your options
- Pre-surgery tests and arrangements

Although the waiting period before your bypass surgery can be stressful for you and your family, it is a good opportunity to learn as much as you can about your operation. Aside from undergoing standard pre-surgery tests, taking the time to understand what you're consenting to and asking your surgeon questions can relieve some of the anxiety you may be feeling. You can also talk about your blood transfusion options at this point.

Meeting Your Cardiac Surgeon

Once you know you are having bypass surgery, you will be referred to a surgeon through your cardiologist to discuss the details of your operation. Most patients will meet with their surgeon only once before the operation, so it's a good idea to come prepared, with a complete medical history and a description of all of your symptoms. Although your surgeon will have already discussed your case with your cardiologist, he or she may ask you for more details. You should also prepare any questions you may have. You may wish to take a family member or friend with you for support.

At this appointment your surgeon should:

- Explain what heart disease means
- Tell you why bypass surgery is the best treatment for your heart disease
- Explain what happens during surgery
- Explain your chances of experiencing complications
- Answer questions
- Talk about what will happen after your surgery
- Give you information about your blood transfusion options (see page 32).

He or she may also ask you to sign a consent form to say that you agree to the operation, as required by law.

Consent

Before you have your bypass surgery, you will need to give your written consent. This is one of the most important steps of your procedure.

What Exactly Is "Consent"?

You make decisions to take risks every day of your life. Some degree of risk is involved when you cross a road, place a bet on a horse, drive your car, or board an airplane. However, when you go into the hospital to have an operation, the risk you take feels different because you are allowing somebody else, usually a doctor, to make decisions for you. Nonetheless, it is a risk just like many other parts of life.

Although the doctor will be acting in your best interest, it is still important that you understand exactly what you are giving your permission for, or consent to. You are therefore entitled to know what is going to happen to you, why you need to have this procedure, what the risks are, and what are the alternatives.

You may be asked for consent for your bypass operation on the day of the procedure or in a pre-admission clinic. It is important that you read the consent form and understand what it is you are signing. Take a few moments to read through it and, if there is enough time, you can take the form home and bring it back on the day of your procedure. If you are worried about any part of the procedure, or you feel you have not received a clear answer on anything, feel free to ask any questions that you may have before signing the form.

"It was not really knowing how long or how difficult the recuperation would be that was frightening."

Ian Gillespie

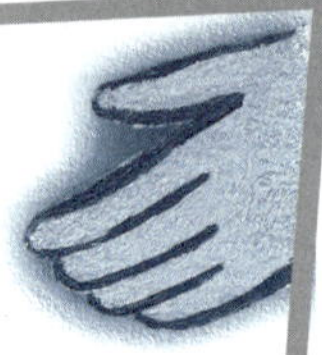

Asking Questions ✓

Here are some questions that you may want to ask before your surgery:

- ○ Why do I need this operation?
- ○ What benefit can I expect from surgery?
- ○ What happens during the procedure?
- ○ What risks are there if I don't have surgery?
- ○ What alternative treatments are available to me?
- ○ Is "beating-heart" surgery an option for me?
- ○ Will you be doing the surgery?
- ○ How many times have you performed this surgery?
- ○ What might go wrong?
- ○ What is my risk of needing a blood transfusion?
- ○ What can I do to reduce the chances of a blood transfusion?
- ○ How long will I be in the hospital?
- ○ How long will I take to recover?

Blood Transfusions

In the early days of bypass surgery, a blood transfusion was inevitable. Nowadays, transfusion is less of an issue for cardiac patients and many patients can avoid a blood transfusion when one or more **blood conservation strategies** (see below) are used before or during surgery. These techniques are included here because some of them need to be planned a few weeks in advance.

Why Is a Transfusion Needed?

Oxygen is carried throughout your body in red blood cells, attached to a protein called **hemoglobin**. If you lose too much blood (around 2 litres or more) during your surgery, your hemoglobin level will fall and your body tissues won't be able to get enough oxygen. This is called **anemia** and can lead to fatigue, a slow recovery, and impaired healing. A transfusion, either of whole blood or specific blood components, such as red cells, can help to prevent this.

How Risky is a Blood Transfusion?

In Canada, a blood transfusion has never been safer. Blood in the blood bank is collected from healthy volunteers by Canadian Blood Services or Héma-Québec and tested for a wide range of viruses, including hepatitis B and C, and HIV. The risk of becoming infected with one of these viruses is now quite small (see Key Point box, page 35). Other common risks of blood transfusions are fever and itchiness, which occur in around 1 in 100 people and are easily treated. Rejection (**hemolytic**) reactions, caused by the incompatibility of the two blood types, can also occur in around 1 in 12,000 people. These are mostly prevented by carrying out a special blood test, called **cross-matching**, before your surgery.

What Are Your Chances of a Transfusion?

Only about 10 percent of first-time bypass patients (1 in 10) need a blood transfusion after an uncomplicated surgery. This can rise to 30 percent or more in longer and more complicated operations. The risk of having a transfusion increases to 50 percent (1 in 2) if this is your second bypass operation or if you are also having a valve operation. Transfusions are about three times more common in women than in men because women have less blood to start with and are also more prone to anemia.

However, the single most important factor in needing a transfusion after surgery is anemia before surgery. This is one of the reasons your blood is tested before surgery, so that you and your physician can correct your anemia before you have your procedure.

Blood Conservation Strategies

Spotting and Treating Anemia

Treating anemia before surgery is one of the most important things you and your physician can do to reduce the chances of a blood transfusion. If your blood tests before surgery show that your hemoglobin is low, your physician may prescribe iron tablets, vitamins (e.g., B12 or folate), or injections of a hormone called **erythropoeitin**. Erythropoetin is naturally secreted by the kidneys to stimulate the body to make more red blood cells and a synthetic version (e.g., Eprex) will gradually correct your anemia by increasing the number of red blood cells in your body. Although it is not common, synthetic erythropoeitin can be used in a heart bypass patient if the physician thinks that it will help him or her.

Blood Banking

One of the best-known blood conservation strategies is blood banking or **autologous blood donation (ABD)**. This involves coming to the clinic several times before your surgery to donate one unit of blood each time. Your blood is stored in the blood bank, reserved for your use, for up to 42 days. If your stored blood is not used by you, it is discarded.

You should talk to your physician at least 3 weeks before your surgery if you are interested in blood banking, but bear in mind it may not be available at your hospital, and it is not possible for many heart-disease patients. Obviously, it is not an option if you need surgery urgently. It is also unsuitable for patients with a recent heart attack, unstable angina, disease in the left main coronary artery, or patients using nitroglycerin patches.

While pre-donating blood may seem an attractive option, it does have a number of disadvantages, and you and your physician should weigh these carefully against its benefits.

Despite careful storage and handling of your pre-donated blood, it will not be exactly the same when you receive it back because of chemical changes during storage. Your pre-donated blood may even become infected with bacteria that will be passed on to you. There is also the small risk of clerical error, so you may end up receiving the wrong blood.

The most important downside to blood banking is that pre-donation—taking your own blood from you—may actually make you anemic before surgery. Anemia is particularly unhealthy for heart patients because their body tissues are already having trouble getting enough oxygen. For this reason, in addition to the inconvenience and discomfort, *pre-donating blood actually increases your risk of receiving a blood transfusion*. One in ten people who pre-donate go on to have a blood transfusion, either of their own blood or from the donor pool.

[KEY POINT]

Donor blood transfusions are potentially life-saving and have never been safer. The risk of HIV infection from donated blood in Canada is now almost one in a million (or 1 in 913,000). By comparison, your risk of dying in a motor-vehicle accident is around 1 in 10,000. Pre-donating blood may seem like a safer option, but in fact it increases your chances of having a blood transfusion—either of your own blood or someone else's—because you may become anemic before surgery.

Acute Normovolemic Hemodilution

The **acute normovolemic hemodilution** technique happens at the time of surgery and is a form of pre-donation. In the operating room, the medical team removes and sets aside 20 to 40 percent of the patient's blood and replaces it with special fluids. This means that any blood lost during the surgical procedure is diluted and contains fewer blood cells. After the surgery, the patient's blood is returned. Clinical trials are currently underway to see whether this technique is helpful for cardiac patients, so you may be offered it.

Cell Salvage

This involves collecting all the blood lost during the operation and returning it to the patient via the heart-lung machine. Various techniques are being tested to find the best way to do this.

Planning Ahead

You should ask your surgeon, anesthesiologist, or both, about your blood conservation options as soon as you know that you are having surgery. If you are anemic, remember that taking your iron tablets as prescribed and eating an iron-rich diet *may* help stave off a blood transfusion. Iron-rich foods include organ meats, turkey and chicken (dark meat), dried fruits, whole grain cereals, peas, beans, and dark green, leafy vegetables (e.g., spinach). You can obtain reliable information on blood conservation from Canadian Blood Services (www.CBS.ca) and Physicians and Nurses for Blood Conservation (www.PNBC.ca).

Home Arrangements

The amount of time you will need off work for your bypass surgery depends on your age and how healthy your heart muscle is. It also depends on how strenuous your occupation is. Generally, you

How Urgent Is My Surgery? [MORE DETAIL]

Not everyone needs surgery right away and some cases are more urgent than others. Your place on the waiting list is decided according to a number of factors:

- The severity of your angina symptoms
- Whether your condition is stable or getting worse
- The amount of medication needed to control your angina
- How badly diseased your arteries are
- The location of your blockage(s)
- Changes in your angina symptoms
- The status of other patients in the system
- Hospital, staff, and equipment availability

NOTIFY YOUR CARDIOLOGIST OR SURGEON if your symptoms change because this may affect your placement on the waiting list.

should plan on taking 6 to 8 weeks off after surgery. Six weeks is about right if you work in an office or have a sedentary job, but you may need 3 months or more if your work is physically demanding.

> "I just wanted to get it over with."
>
> **Mel Isen**

Some patients like to sort out financial loose ends and other paperwork before surgery. Some patients also like to draw up a "living will." A living will clearly informs your family and your physician about exactly what treatment you would like and, probably more importantly, would *not* like, in the event that you fall into a coma. You may not wish to pursue this; it's just something to think about.

Pre-admission Clinics

Unless your surgery was an urgent or emergency procedure, you may be offered a pre-admission class 1 or 2 weeks before being admitted to the hospital for surgery. This 1-hour class gives you the opportunity to meet members of your surgical team and ask them questions. The hospital will encourage family members to come along, too, because families play a key role in recovery. There may be a short video about what to expect before, during, and after surgery, your recovery in the hospital and at home, and personal accounts of patients who have had heart bypass surgery.

On the day of your pre-admission class, you may also meet an anesthesiologist, and get some blood tests and a chest X-ray. These tests are important because they allow your doctor to check whether your health has changed significantly since he or she last saw you. They also give a point of comparison for tests that will be carried out after your operation.

If you cannot attend a pre-admission class—because, for instance, you live out of town—you will probably be told to come to the hospital the day before your surgery to allow these tests to be done.

Meeting Your Anesthesiologist

You may meet an anesthesiologist at your pre-admission clinic or right before your surgery. He or she is an important part of your health-care team before, during, and after surgery. The anesthesiologist's role is to take a full medical history from you, decide which anesthetic is best for you during your surgery, and make decisions about blood conservation and transfusion. This individual will not necessarily be the same person who puts you to sleep in the operating room, but you can ask about any concerns that you may have. The anesthesiologist will also review your medications and give you advice about which should be stopped before surgery.

Blood Tests

Your blood is tested to measure red and white blood cell counts and check how your liver, kidneys, and hormone glands are working. Blood sugar and cholesterol levels may also be checked so that they can be compared before and after surgery.

Chest X-ray

This is a routine test to check for lung congestion, respiratory disease, or heart-chamber enlargement. If your X-ray shows a problem, you may be referred to a lung specialist (**pulmonologist**) for further testing before your surgery.

[SELF-HELP]

When to Call Your Doctor

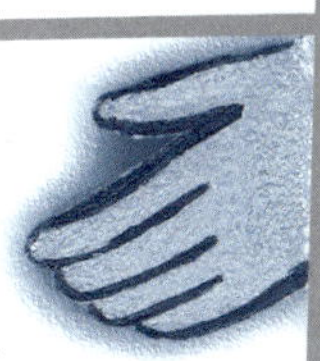

While you are waiting for your surgery, tell your doctor if :

- Your existing symptoms become worse or more frequent
- Your symptoms occur at rest or at night
- You need more nitroglycerine to relieve chest pain
- Your chest discomfort comes on more quickly and lasts longer
- You notice new symptoms, such as heart palpitations, a fast heart rate, an irregular heart beat, or shortness of breath
- You gain more than 2.5 kg (5 lbs) in 1 week and have swollen ankles or hands
- You generally feel worse since you last visited your doctor

IF YOU EXPERIENCE ANGINA LASTING LONGER THAN 15 to 20 MINUTES, WHICH IS NOT RELIEVED BY THREE DOSES OF NITROGLYCERINE, CALL 911 TO TAKE YOU TO THE NEAREST HOSPITAL.

Electrocardiogram (ECG)

By the time you reach this point, you should be familiar with an ECG, the most commonly used test to check on heart function. In this test, soft plastic electrodes attached to your chest, arms, and legs are connected to a machine that records your heart's electrical activity.

What Happens Next?

Once you have attended the pre-admission clinic, the next step is the surgery itself.

Chapter 5

the day of your bypass surgery

What Happens in this Chapter

- Your hospital checklist
- Medicines before surgery
- The night before surgery
- Arrival at the hospital
- Preparations for your surgery

You will be admitted to the hospital early on the actual day of your surgery unless you need some extra tests, in which case you will be asked to arrive the day before. Remember to leave your valuables at home and bring all your medications with you. You should not eat or drink after midnight on the day before your procedure, or your surgery may be canceled. Once in the hospital, your care team will get you ready for your surgery and you will be transferred to the operating room as soon as it becomes available.

Planning Your Day

Here are a few tips to help you plan your hospital visit.

- Do not to eat or drink anything after midnight the night before your surgery.
- Sips of water are fine if you need to take medication.
- Avoid caffeine and alcohol.
- Try to get a good night's rest.
- If you have trouble sleeping the night before your surgery, try the following:
  - Relaxation techniques (see page 114)
  - Herbal tea (decaffeinated)
  - Talking about your concerns to loved ones
  - A sedative prescribed by your doctor
- Prepare your skin, as you were instructed at your pre-admission class, by showering with antiseptic soap the night before and in the morning.
- Don't shave body hair. Your hair will be clipped by one of the nurses in the hospital to decrease the chance of infection.
- Don't forget to take the suppository from your preparation package the night before to avoid constipation after your operation.

Packing Your Bag for the Hospital

The hospital is a busy place. Your care team won't necessarily have the time or resources to provide you with everything you need during your hospital stay. There are a number of items that you should bring with you to the hospital and some that you should leave at home.

Comfortable clothing

Immediately after surgery, while you are in the intensive care unit, you will be in a hospital gown. However, once you are transferred from the intensive care unit to the patient ward, you may prefer to wear your own pajamas, sweat suit, or robe. You will be walking around the patient unit and transported for tests, so you are likely to be most comfortable in your own clothes. Slippers are a good idea, as well as a supportive pair of shoes for exercising later in your recovery. If you can, take shoes or slippers that are one size larger than usual because your feet may swell after surgery. Women may find that a front-opening bra is more comfortable than one that opens at the back.

Your Own Pillow and Pillowcase

Sleep loss is one of the most common problems that patients have to deal with after surgery. Sometimes the smallest comforts from home can make a difference in how well you progress while you're in the hospital. Your own pillow can help you feel more comfortable during the day and sleep more restfully at night.

Personal Items

You won't be provided with toiletries, so be sure to pack your own items such as toothbrush, toothpaste, hairbrush or comb, deodorant, razor, or shaving cream. Write your name on any containers for prosthetics such as dentures, hearing aids, contact lenses, or corrective glasses. Because you will be asked to remove any prostheses just before you are taken to the operating room, it is important that these items be well-marked to ensure they are returned to you. You may even want to give them to a family member for safekeeping.

Activities

It is normal for your attention span to be short or for you to have difficulty concentrating while recovering. Consider renting a TV and bring simple activities such as magazines or books with lots of pictures, knitting, crossword puzzles, or playing cards for solitaire, and small amounts of cash for candy or gum from the hospital shop. It's best to leave any personal or professional work at home. At this point, it is important that you focus your energy on your health and recovery.

Leave Valuables at Home

Leave valuables such as rings, jewelry, watches, wallet, purse, cell phone, laptop, credit cards, or large amounts of cash at home. Unfortunately, there have been situations in every hospital where items have been misplaced, lost, or even stolen.

What Should I Do about my Medicines?

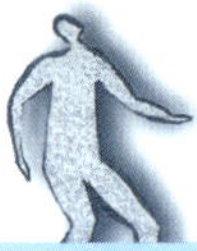

[MORE DETAIL]

- Continue taking your medications right up until surgery unless your doctor tells you otherwise.
- Make sure you are given specific instructions for each of your medications at the pre-admission clinic. Do not forget to mention vitamins, herbs, etc., in your medication list.
- Normally, blood thinners such as Coumadin and Aspirin are stopped a few days before surgery, but be guided by your physician.
- If you are taking steroids your surgeon may reduce your dosage.
- Bring all your medication bottles, or a list of them, to the hospital when you are admitted *whether or not you are currently taking them.*

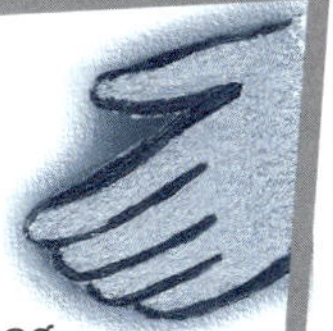

Hospital Checklist ✓

You may find this checklist useful as you pack your bag.

- ○ All your medicines in their original bottles or a list of them
- ○ Comfortable clothing, e.g., sweat suit, front-opening bra
- ○ Slippers
- ○ Supportive shoes
- ○ Your own pillow and pillowcase
- ○ Toiletry bag
- ○ Dentures, glasses, hearing aids marked with your name
- ○ Reading materials
- ○ Other activities, e.g., pack of cards, crosswords
- ○ Small amount of cash
- ○ Phone numbers of friends and family

Leave behind:

- ○ Valuables, e.g., wallet, jewelry, cell phone
- ○ Work

Hospital Admission

You may be admitted to the hospital the day of or the day before your surgery—this will be decided by your surgeon. Many patients who are admitted the day before need a "work-up," which means that you need to be seen by a doctor from another specialty, e.g., **nephrology**, if you have a history of kidney failure, or **endocrinology**, if you are diabetic with poor blood-sugar control.

If you are admitted the day before your surgery, a nurse will talk to you about preparing for your operation and give you a suppository to help you have a bowel movement.

If you are admitted to the hospital on the day of your surgery, you will need to arrive at the hospital early in the morning, having had nothing to eat or drink since midnight the night before, and proceed to the **pre-admission area**. A nurse will greet you and show you to a room where you will be instructed to shower with antiseptic soap, go to the bathroom, if necessary, and change into a hospital gown and cap. You should have already taken a suppository at home the night before, but if it didn't work, you will be given another one.

The nurse will then clip your chest and leg hair using sterile scissors. You may be given a sedative in the form of a needle or pill that will make you feel drowsy or relaxed. A hospital attendant will then take you to the surgical area on a stretcher. Be sure to make yourself comfortable; ask for extra pillows or blankets if necessary. The wait in this area may be 10 to 30 minutes. During this time, the staff will continue to keep you updated about when you will proceed to the operating room. The anesthesiologist may introduce him or herself at this point if you have not previously met. He or she will have already reviewed your notes and be very familiar with your case (see page 38).

"The time passed and I read and I talked to people on the phone, and I pretty well tried to carry on a relatively normal day."

Mel Isen

What Happens Next?

After your preparation for surgery is complete, you will go into the operating room. The anesthesiologist will put you to sleep very quickly and your operation will begin. The next two chapters tell you about what will happen during your surgery. If you'd rather not know the details of your operation, turn to Chapter 8, "When It's All Over," to find out what to expect immediately after surgery.

Chapter 6

the coronary bypass procedure

What Happens in this Chapter

- A step-by-step guide to your coronary bypass
- The general anesthetic
- Types of bypass graft
- The heart-lung machine
- The grafting procedure
- Closing the incision

Coronary artery bypass grafting has been around for over 30 years. Although it may seem scary, the idea is surprisingly simple. To restore blood flow to the muscle of the heart, the blocked coronary artery is bypassed using a blood vessel taken from elsewhere in the body. There are many variations on this basic strategy. The heart may be kept beating or briefly stopped. The graft may be a vein or an artery, and it may be removed entirely from its original position or remain anchored at one end. Your surgeon will advise you which options are open to you, based on your medical history. Even though you may not be able to choose which route your surgery will take, this chapter will help you understand the alternatives before giving permission for your surgery to go ahead.

What Is Bypass Surgery?

The technical term for heart bypass surgery is **coronary artery bypass graft (CABG) surgery**. It aims to restore blood flow to your heart by attaching, or grafting, one or more new veins or arteries onto your coronary arteries below the level of the blockage (see Figures 6–2 and 6–3). **Saphenous veins** (from the leg) or arteries such as the **radial** (from the arm) or **internal thoracic arteries** (from the chest wall) are commonly used as grafts.

It is important to realize that because the coronary arteries are on the surface of the heart, the grafts will be attached to the outside of your heart. Unless you are having valve surgery, the surgeon will not open up your heart at all, except to insert tubes for the connection to the heart-lung machine.

The traditional coronary artery bypass procedure takes 4 to 6 hours and involves opening the front of the chest by making a vertical cut in the breastbone (or **sternum**) and then gently pulling aside the ribs to expose the heart. After the patient is connected to a heart-lung machine, which takes over the job of pumping blood around the body during the operation, the heart is gradually stopped and the surgery can proceed. A vein or an artery, or both, that have been carefully removed from elsewhere in the body are sewn into place on the outside of the heart. The heart is then restarted, the heart-lung machine is disconnected, the chest wall is closed, and you are ready to leave the operating room (see More Detail box on page 50).

There are variations on this traditional approach. In some circumstances and in some hospitals, surgeons are operating on the beating heart, to avoid the side effects of the heart-lung machine. This is called **beating-heart surgery,** or **off-pump surgery (OPCAB)**. Another technique, called **minimally invasive heart surgery (MIDCAB)**, in which the surgeon enters the chest through small incisions between the ribs, is also an option, although it is uncommon. These approaches are discussed in more detail in Chapter 7. The current chapter will discuss traditional bypass surgery.

Whichever method your surgical team uses, the goals of your coronary bypass surgery are the same:

- To improve blood flow to your heart muscle
- To relieve your angina symptoms
- To improve your quality of life
- To keep the risks of surgery to a minimum
- To prolong your life.

Getting Ready

When you are brought into the operating room (see Figure 6–1), you will be introduced to a technician who will help you up onto the operating table. The table is quite narrow, so you may feel more secure if you feel for both sides of the table to ensure that you are in the middle. There will always be someone there to help and support you.

The operating room will be busy with nurses, technicians, the anesthesiologist, and, possibly, one or more resident surgeons (see Chapter 14). The staffing arrangements will vary from hospital to hospital. You may not see the surgeon immediately before your surgery because at this point he or she will be reviewing your chart and angiogram films. Staff will be wearing special sterile uniforms (scrubs) and head coverings, as well as masks and gloves.

One of the first things you may notice is the temperature of the

Your Coronary Bypass Procedure [MORE DETAIL]

These are the basic steps of traditional CABG surgery. If this is all the detail you can handle right now, you may wish to skip to Chapter 8 once you have finished reading this box.

1. Monitors are connected to you, e.g., ECG pads, blood-pressure cuff.
2. Plastic tubes are inserted into an artery and a vein in your arm, under local anesthetic. The tube in the artery measures blood pressure, the venous line is for giving medications and fluids.
3. An oxygen mask is placed over your mouth and nose and you are asked to breathe normally.
4. You are given a general anesthetic—probably through the intravenous line (not the oxygen mask).
5. Once you are asleep, you are attached to the breathing machine (ventilator).
6. Other monitors and tubes are attached to you as needed.
7. You are washed with antiseptic and covered with sterile drapes.
8. Your chest is opened along the breastbone.
9. Your grafts are removed from elsewhere in your body (e.g., the arms or legs, and put aside).
10. You are connected to the heart-lung machine.
11. Your heart is stopped and cooled.
12. Grafts are attached to the outside of your heart.
13. Your heart is warmed and restarted.
14. The heart-lung machine is turned off and the ventilator breathes for you once again.
15. The heart-lung tubes are removed from your heart.
16. Drainage tubes are placed in your chest to measure bleeding after the surgery.
17. Temporary pacemaker wires are placed on the surface of your heart.
18. Your breastbone is closed with permanent stainless steel wires.
19. Tissue above the breastbone is closed with dissolving stitches.
20. You leave the operating room still asleep, connected to the ventilator.

room. The temperature is deliberately kept low for comfort and to allow cooling of your body.

While the surgical team is busy preparing for your operation, you may have time to look around. There will be a certain amount of noise, such as beeping machines and people talking or moving about doing their jobs. This is all normal preparation for your surgery.

Large round lights above the table give the surgeon good lighting for your operation. At the head of the bed you will see the large anesthetic machine that the anesthesiologist will use throughout the procedure. Another large piece of equipment that may be off to the side of the room is the **cardiopulmonary bypass machine** (or **heart-lung machine**) that your team will use later in the surgery (see page 61).

Figure 6–1. The Operating Room (OR)

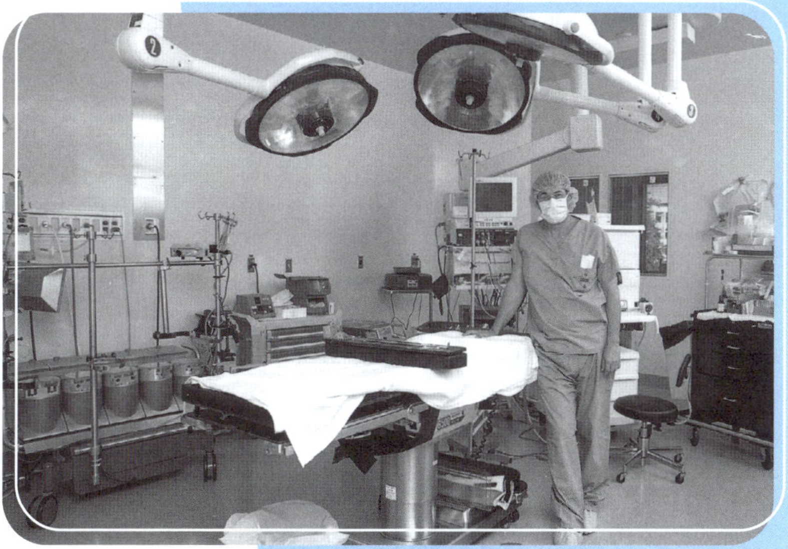

This is where you will have your heart surgery.

> "Going there I was scared, very frightened. But when I got in, they worked pretty fast. I remember them transferring me from the stretcher onto the table and then after that, several seconds later, I was out."
>
> **Mel Isen**

Once you are lying comfortably, you will be covered with a blanket and positioned so that both arms are outstretched, out of the way of your chest. You will then be attached to a number of monitors that will let your team keep an eye on your progress during the procedure. The round sticky pads of the ECG (heart monitor) and blood-pressure cuff will already be familiar to you. Additionally, a small clip called a **pulse oximeter** will be placed on either your ear or finger. This is used to measure the amount of oxygen in your blood.

Next, the team will insert two narrow tubes into your forearm—one into a vein (an **intravenous line** or **IV**) and one into an artery (an **arterial line**). The IV line is used to give drugs and fluid, and the arterial line is used for blood sampling and providing beat-by-beat blood-pressure monitoring. You won't be aware of this, but a **Foley catheter** will also be inserted after you are asleep to empty your bladder and closely monitor your urine output during surgery.

The General Anesthetic

When the monitors and lines are in place you are ready for your general anesthetic. An assistant will place an oxygen mask over your mouth and nose and you will be asked to breathe normally.

A general anesthetic is not one drug but a cocktail of medications—each with different roles. It includes drugs to put you to sleep (**induction drugs**), vapor drugs to keep you asleep, and muscle relaxants. For more on anesthetics, see Chapter 12. From the time a general anesthetic starts, patients rarely have any recall of

[SELF-HELP]

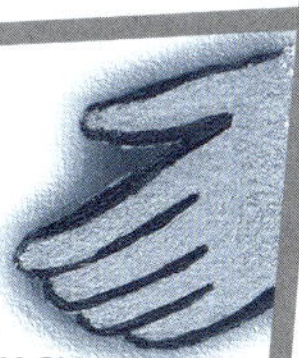

The oxygen mask

The oxygen mask often has a plastic-like smell, or it may be scented to cover this odor. Be assured that, unless your anesthesiologist tells you otherwise, the strange smell is not the anesthetic vapor. Most people receive a general anesthetic through an IV line.

events and 70 percent of patients do not remember entering the operating room. Your anesthesiologist can precisely control your level of consciousness and will take you from being wide awake to deep surgical anesthesia in a matter of moments.

The risks of general anesthesia are carefully managed using an array of sophisticated monitors and your anesthesiologist will watch you carefully throughout the surgery. The dangers of a general anesthetic are now just a small part of the overall risks of bypass surgery.

How Do They Know I'm Asleep?

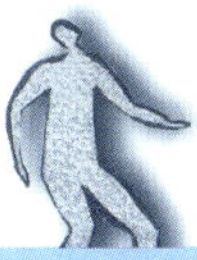

[MORE DETAIL]

Many people fear that they might wake up or be aware during surgery. This is very rare, especially in pre-planned cardiac surgery, which involves a deep level of anesthesia. It happens in fewer than 3 in 1,000 operations, and when it does happen, most patients describe the memory as brief, vague, and painless.

Final Preparations

Once you are asleep, your anesthesiologist will carefully place a tube down your windpipe. This is attached to a breathing machine (ventilator) that will breathe for you during surgery. He or she will then place an additional IV line in your neck called the **central venous pressure (CVP)** line. This line provides access for a specialized monitor called the **pulmonary artery (PA) catheter**, which gives detailed information about your blood pressure and heart activity. Not everyone needs a PA catheter, but the CVP line is always put in place just in case the information from a PA catheter is needed.

Finally, a plastic tube may be inserted through your nose and into your stomach to prevent nausea or vomiting when you wake up after surgery.

Once all your lines and tubes are in place, and your team is confident that they can follow your progress every step of the way, they will cleanse your body from neck to foot with an antiseptic solution.

The surgical team will then cover your body with sterile drapes. These drapes are used to create what surgeons call the **sterile field**. They will cover your entire body surface except for the areas that need to be exposed for the procedure, such as your chest and your arm or leg.

Two things now happen at the same time. While one surgical team carefully prepares all the arteries and veins that will be used as grafts in your bypass surgery, a second team prepares your heart to receive these grafts. These parts of the operation will be described one after another, but in reality they are happening simultaneously.

Preparing Your Heart

Most coronary artery bypass procedures involve making a neat cut down the middle of the breastbone (**sternum**) from just below the neck to the lower part of the chest. The length of your own incision will depend on your anatomy and build. The breastbone is divided using a special power saw and any bleeding is quickly controlled using an **electrocautery device** (see Glossary). The edges of the breastbone are then carefully lifted up and outward, and held in place using a device called a **retractor**. This gives the surgeon a good view of the heart and the thoracic arteries, if these are being used as grafts (see page 57). The protective sac around the heart (the **pericardium**) is then opened to give your surgeon access to your coronary arteries, which lie on the surface of the heart.

Preparing Your Grafts

During coronary artery bypass graft surgery, as the name implies, your blocked coronary arteries will be bypassed using your own blood vessels taken from elsewhere in the body and grafted onto your heart. Selecting the best **bypass graft** or **conduit** for each coronary artery is one of the most important decisions that your surgeon will make and he or she will choose grafts that are going to give you the best chance of a successful result.

An ideal graft is free of disease or blockage itself and is a good size match for the artery to be bypassed. Another important consideration for your surgeon is how long the chosen graft is likely to stay open, or free from blockage—this is called the **patency** (see More Detail box on page 56). Grafts from arteries (**arterial grafts**) are used whenever possible since these are less likely to block up in the future. Although your surgeon will discuss your options with you beforehand, the type of graft is often determined by your medical circumstances. **Vein grafts** may be needed for some people or some types of bypass (see page 60). Your surgeon will decide which grafts are best for you.

A "standard" triple bypass consists of an **internal thoracic artery graft** (see Figure 6–2) and two **vein bypasses** (see Figure 6–3).

After the artery or vein is removed from its original site, it is gently wrapped in a chemically soaked sponge until it is needed. The incision in the arm or leg is then sewn closed using either stitches that dissolve on their own or staples that will need to be removed after you are discharged from the hospital.

How Long do Bypass Grafts Last?

[MORE DETAIL]

Type of Graft	**Still Open**	
	1 year after surgery	10 years after surgery
Vein	85 to 90%	40 to 60%
Internal thoracic artery	95 to 100%	80 to 95%
Radial artery	88 to 97%	89% at 5 years (10 years not known yet)

Bear in mind that these are not hard-and-fast predictions. These studies were carried out several years ago, on patients who are different from you. Improved surgical techniques and medications mean that success rates are probably much higher now.

Internal Thoracic Artery Graft

The thoracic arteries, also known as the mammary arteries, are a popular choice for bypass grafts in many patients. They run down the underside of the chest wall. Your surgeon may leave one end of the thoracic artery where it is, and graft the cut end onto your heart

Figure 6–2. Thoracic Artery Graft

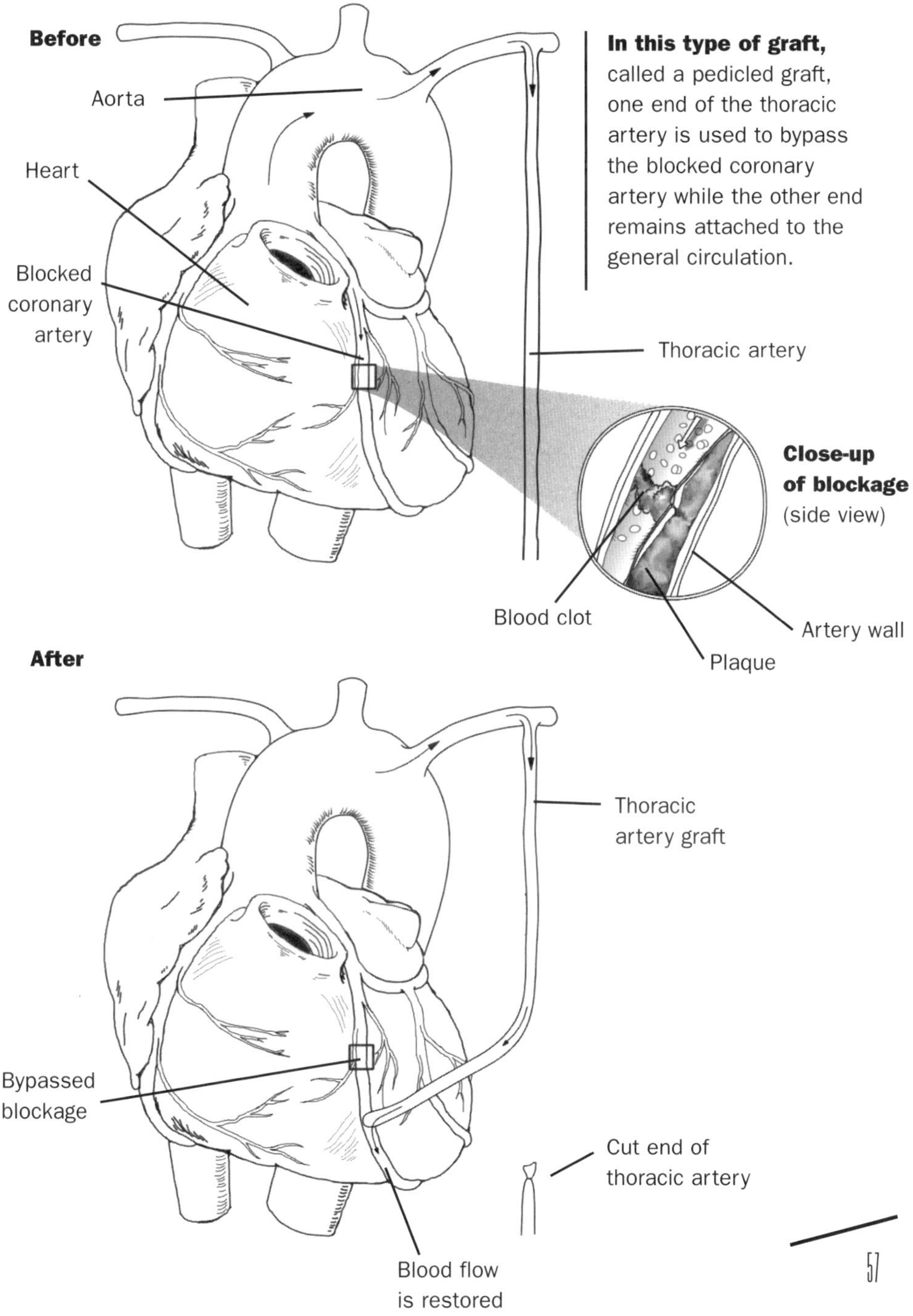

In this type of graft, called a pedicled graft, one end of the thoracic artery is used to bypass the blocked coronary artery while the other end remains attached to the general circulation.

(a pedicled graft, see Figure 6–2), or remove it completely and create a free graft.

The main advantage of internal thoracic artery grafts is their excellent long-term results (see More Detail box on page 56). The downside of these grafts is that they are more difficult and time-consuming to get at than other grafts (because they are in the chest), so they may be unsuitable in emergency surgery. They are also not suitable for people with certain medical conditions, such as respiratory disease. Recovery may also be more uncomfortable: some patients experience numbness or tingling in the chest wall. However, this subsides with time.

Radial Artery Graft

The **radial artery** runs down your forearm, parallel to the long bones. Before the radial can be used for a graft, your medical team will need to check that the other major artery in the arm (the **ulnar**) can provide adequate blood flow to the hand by performing a simple test called the **Allen's test** (see Glossary). If this is not the case, a radial artery graft is not possible.

[KEY POINT]

If you have had varicose veins or vein stripping, be sure to tell your surgeon before surgery. This will affect which veins he or she chooses as grafts. Superficial spider veins, however, are usually not a problem.

To remove the radial artery, the surgeon will make a cut along the inside of the arm from just below the elbow to the wrist. The artery is then snipped at each end and gently lifted clear of the arm (see Figure 6–3).

The radial artery is a good choice for a graft because it is long, easy to get at, and has good long-term results (see More Detail box, page 56). The disadvantages of this kind of graft are that your arm will be sore and swollen

Figure 6–3. Radial Artery and Vein Grafts

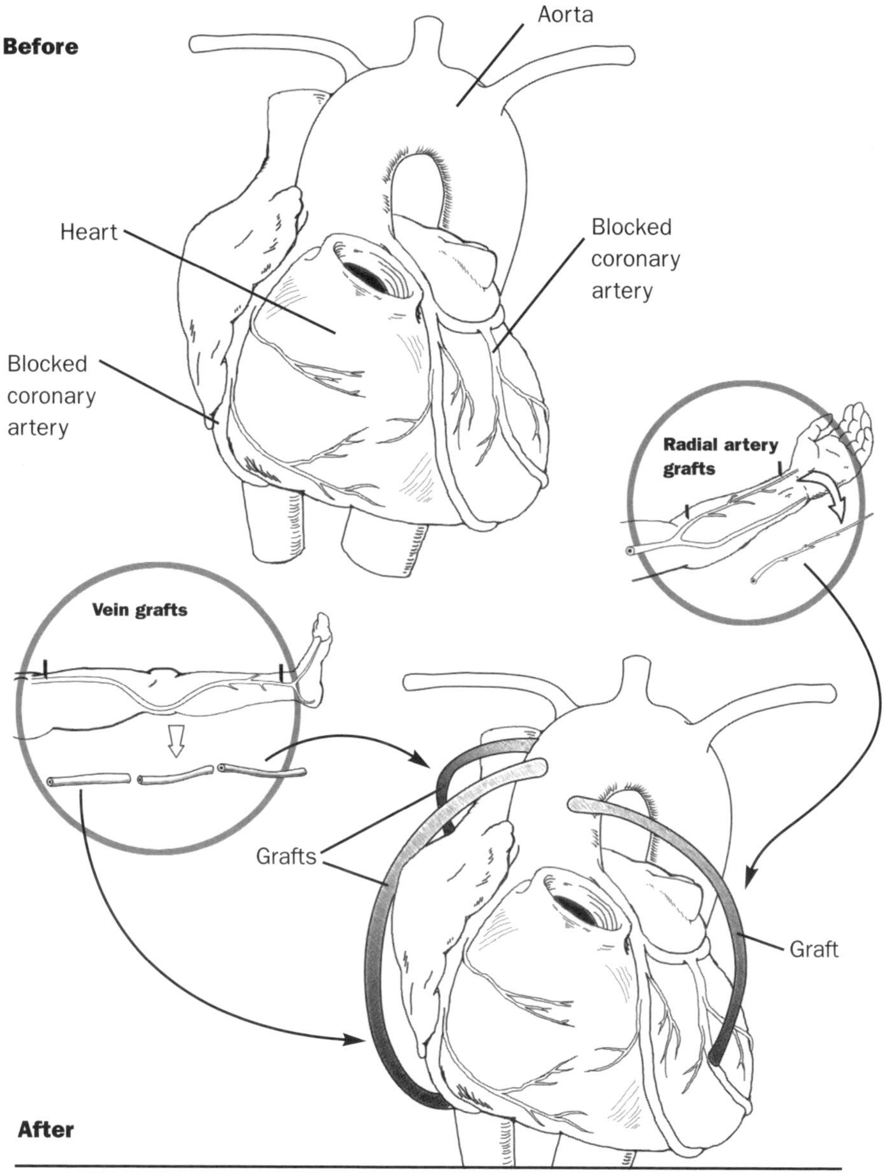

Radial and vein grafts are created from the radial artery in the arm or the saphenous vein in the leg. The artery or vein is divided into smaller sections, which are then used to bypass the blocked coronary arteries.

> "I said to the doctor 3 days after the operation, 'You didn't tell me you were doing five [arteries]. You said you were going to do three.' He sort of laughed and said, 'Well, we were going to wake you up, but we decided not to. We just went ahead and did them.'"
>
> **Jim Morning**

afterwards, and fine motor control may be permanently affected. This means that this type of graft is not suitable for people with hobbies or professions that involve fine motor control, and is also why the non-dominant hand is used. The radial artery is also prone to spasm, so you may need to take medicines such as **calcium channel blockers** for 3 to 6 months after your surgery to stop this from happening.

Leg (Saphenous) Vein Graft

Your **saphenous vein** starts on the top of your foot and ends near your groin. It is usually removed through an incision the length of your leg (see Figure 6–3). Some surgeons use **minimally invasive** surgery to extract the vein through a smaller cut.

The main advantage of a vein graft is that it is very quick and the vein is very easy to get at—useful during emergency surgery. Vein grafts are also a better option than arterial grafts for certain kinds of patients. You are more likely to have a vein graft if you are over 80 years old or have one of the following medical conditions:

- Need urgent bypass surgery
- Need other heart surgery
- Unstable angina/recent heart attack
- Inadequate radial or internal thoracic arteries
- Extensive previous chest surgery
- Another serious illness, e.g., cancer, diabetes, lung disease, kidney failure
- Blood disorder, e.g., anemia
- Obesity

The downside of vein grafts is that they are more likely to block up than arterial grafts (see page 56), although the long-term picture can be improved by controlling risk factors such as cigarette smoking, high blood pressure, diabetes, and high cholesterol. Additionally, vein grafts may not be an option if you have varicose or stripped veins, or poor circulation generally. For these, and other, reasons vein grafts are increasingly uncommon in younger patients.

Heart-Lung Machine

Once the grafts for the bypass are prepared, the surgeon and the anesthesiologist will work together with a specialized technician called a **perfusionist** to connect you to the **cardiopulmonary bypass (CPB)**, or **heart-lung**, machine. The reason that the heart-lung machine is used in traditional bypass surgery is to allow the surgeon to work on a heart that is not beating. This obviously makes surgery much easier. The heart-lung machine takes over the job of oxygenating the blood and pumping it around the body while the heart is stopped (see Figure 6–4).

Figure 6–4. The Heart-Lung Machine

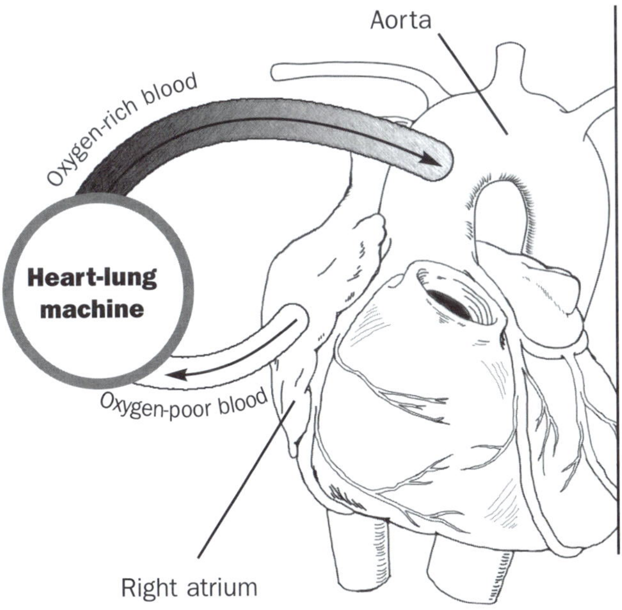

This machine takes over the roles of the heart and the lungs during bypass surgery. The patient is connected to the machine through two tubes inserted into the heart. The tube from the right atrium carries oxygen-poor blood out of the body into the heart-lung machine. The tube to the aorta carries newly oxygenated blood from the machine back into the body.

Once the heart-lung machine takes over, the heart is stopped by a process called **cardioplegia**. This involves treating the heart with a chemical solution that temporarily stops the heart-muscle fibers from contracting. Once the heart stops moving, the bypass grafts can be attached.

Attaching the Grafts

Your surgeon will bypass all significantly blocked coronary arteries unless they are too small (less than 1.5mm in diameter) or the blocked arteries supply heart muscle that is already scarred or damaged due to a heart attack. Three to five bypasses are placed during an average procedure. The number that you receive will depend on how many blocked arteries you have, and how important they are.

In order to connect the graft to the coronary artery, your surgeon will make an opening in the coronary artery just beyond the blockage. One end of the graft is then fixed into place over the opening with fine stitches (**sutures**). The other end of the graft is connected to the aorta—or even to another graft (see Figure 6–3). Once the grafts are in place, blood will be able to bypass the areas of blockage.

If you are having a pedicled thoracic artery graft (see Figure 6–2), the free end of the artery that was removed from the chest wall will be sewn into one of your coronary arteries at a point beyond the blockage, while the other end will remain attached to the general circulation.

Coronary Endarterectomy

In some patients, the coronary artery beyond the blockage is too diseased to receive a graft and there are other blockages further downstream, in which case the surgeon may opt to clean out the

Pacemaker Wires

[MORE DETAIL]

After surgery, the heart can need electrical stimulation to help it beat, so your surgeon may implant fine wires into the heart that can be attached to an external pacemaker if required. You will see the wires protruding through your skin. They will be removed once your heart rate and rhythm return to normal.

coronary artery before placing the grafts. This procedure, called **endarterectomy**, involves stripping out the diseased material from the inside of the coronary artery and has been likened to a robin pulling a worm from the ground.

Blood Conservation

Throughout your procedure, your surgical team will be using one or more techniques to reduce the amount of blood that you lose, recycle blood that you do lose, and reduce the chances that you will need a blood transfusion. These **blood conservation** techniques are discussed in more detail in Chapter 4.

Final Stages

Once the bypasses are attached and the procedure is complete, the surgeon, perfusionist, and anesthesiologist will all work together to disconnect you from the heart-lung machine.

About 30 minutes before the end of the procedure, the surgeon will ask the perfusionist to start rewarming the circulating blood in the heart-lung machine. As your heart warms up, it will start to beat spontaneously. Your team will gradually wean you off the heart-lung machine by slowly decreasing the amount of blood diverted into the machine. When your heart is beating strongly on its own and your blood pressure is stable, the heart-lung machine will be turned off and the ventilator will start breathing for you again. The tubes connecting you to the heart-lung machine will then be removed from your heart.

Next, drainage tubes will be placed in the spaces between the lungs and the rib cage and in front of the heart. These tubes will remain in place for a day or two to drain any excess fluid from around your surgery site. The breastbone will then be closed with permanent stainless steel wires. Once you are healed you will not be aware of these wires, which are completely inert and do not need to be removed. They will show up on chest X-rays but have no effect on metal detectors. Finally, the tissue above the breastbone will be closed with stitches that dissolve on their own.

What Happens Next?

Once the heart-lung machine is discontinued and the incisions are closed, your surgical team will want to keep a close eye on you for a few hours, so your next stop is the **intensive care unit (ICU)**. Chapter 8 tells you what to expect when you wake up to the greeting of a nurse in the cardiovascular ICU.

Chapter 7

non-traditional bypass surgery

What Happens in this Chapter

- Traditional versus "beating-heart" surgery
- Disadvantages of the heart-lung machine
- Pros and cons of traditional versus non-traditional approaches
- A step-by-step guide to off-pump and minimally invasive surgery

Before the arrival of the heart-lung machine in the 1960s, all heart surgery took place on a moving, beating heart. Technology has now come full circle, and once again surgeons are operating on the beating heart, this time to avoid the side effects of the heart-lung machine. There are a number of ways to do this—some are more successful than others, and some are only suitable for certain kinds of patients. As with all medical treatments, there are no easy answers and you will have to weigh the risks and benefits of these procedures with your surgeon before deciding whether non-traditional bypass surgery is right for you.

What is Non-Traditional Bypass Surgery?

> "We're very fortunate to have the doctors and the hospitals that we have, and the medical technology that we have today that wasn't available years ago."
>
> **Marie McVety**

As described in Chapter 6, traditional coronary artery bypass surgery involves stopping the heart and using a heart-lung machine to pump blood around the body during surgery. Non-traditional bypass surgery is any procedure in which the heart continues to beat during surgery and the heart-lung machine is not used. For this reason, it is also known as **beating-heart surgery**. The aim of this kind of surgery is to avoid problems associated with the heart-lung machine (see page 23) and provide an option for patients with less severe heart disease.

There are a number of challenges involved in operating on a beating heart. Apart from the practical difficulty that it is hard to stitch a moving object, it is also more difficult to get at the blood vessels at the back of the heart, such as sections of the right coronary artery. Therefore, beating-heart surgery is not suitable for everyone. Another general consideration, if you are offered beating-heart surgery, is that traditional bypass surgery has a very long history, the techniques are well practiced, and the results are well-known for a wide variety of patients. This is not true for non-traditional techniques, which are still evolving.

Over the years, a variety of methods have been developed to improve the results of beating-heart surgery. In this chapter we describe the most common techniques: basic **off-pump coronary artery bypass (OPCAB)** surgery and **minimally invasive direct coronary artery bypass (MIDCAB)** surgery. Some surgeons also combine MIDCAB with angioplasty (**hybrid procedure**), which is not discussed here.

Off-Pump (OPCAB) Surgery

The preparations for OPCAB are similar to those for traditional bypass surgery (Chapter 6), and the chest is opened in a similar way. However, the heart is not stopped and the heart-lung bypass is not used, although a heart-lung machine will be on standby in case the OPCAB is not successful. To reduce bleeding, just before the grafts are attached, a gentle tourniquet is applied to the upper end of the coronary artery that is going to be bypassed. The whole area is then stabilized with a fork-like instrument, while an assistant keeps the surgical site dry with a small blower.

The heart muscle can survive for up to 30 minutes without blood flow, so there is plenty of time to attach the grafts before the tourniquet needs to be removed. In the unlikely event that your heartbeat starts to falter, you will be connected to a heart-lung machine to maintain circulation around your body.

Advantages of Off-Pump Surgery

There are not many studies directly comparing the advantages of OPCAB versus traditional bypass surgery, because OPCAB is still fairly new. Studies so far show that a blood transfusion is less likely in OPCAB—a plus for those who do not accept blood products. Some patients are able to have chest tubes removed more quickly afterward, and are able to leave the hospital earlier. Off-pump surgery may cause fewer cognitive side effects (impaired memory or concentration) than traditional CABG because early studies show that there are fewer microscopic brain changes after off-pump surgery than traditional surgery. However, off-pump surgery does not seem to reduce patients' risk of having a stroke.

Disdvantages of Off-Pump Surgery

The main concern about off-pump surgery is that we do not yet know the long-term success rates of the technique. Because it is more difficult to attach a graft to a beating heart, these grafts may have a shorter life than grafts performed on a non-beating heart. It is also not for everyone. Off-pump surgery appears to work best for carefully selected patients. These include patients with blockages in the left coronary artery or the top part of the right coronary artery, those who need only a small number of grafts, those who are at high risk of having a stroke, have disease in the main artery of the body (the aorta), or have kidney problems. Also bear in mind that off-pump surgery does not guarantee that you will avoid the heart-lung machine. You may need it after all if your heart does not respond well to the procedure.

Minimally Invasive Bypass (MIDCAB) Surgery

MIDCAB, or "keyhole heart surgery," is another technique in which the heart is beating during surgery and the heart-lung machine is not used. The surgeon is able to get at the heart through one or more small incisions between the ribs under the left breast. Your surgeon may use a small camera to see the heart (**thoracoscopy**) or the incision may be made a little larger and your heart observed directly. MIDCAB is most successful for blockages in the left anterior descending artery and the graft is always the internal thoracic artery (page 56).

The preparations for MIDCAB are similar to those for traditional bypass surgery (Chapter 6) and, in fact, you will be fully prepared for traditional surgery from top to toe in case your surgeon decides that MIDCAB is not possible.

If the surgeon decides to go ahead with MIDCAB, but is not using thoracoscopy, he or she will then place a special clamp called a **retractor** to hold the incision open and give a good view of the heart and thoracic artery. If you are having thoracoscopy, the surgeon will make three more small incisions between your ribs to allow the camera and the instruments to be inserted into your chest. Once the procedure is complete, the instruments will be removed and the incision will be closed with sutures or staples.

Minimally Invasive Bypass Surgery—Is It Right for You? [MORE DETAIL]

You are more likely to be a candidate for MIDCAB if you have one or more of these factors:

- Blockage in one or (at the most) two accessible arteries in the left side of the heart that cannot be treated with angioplasty
- Other chronic illness, such as a recent stroke, uncontrolled diabetes, kidney disease, or a blood disorder
- Aged over 75 years
- Normal **left ventricular function** (see Glossary)
- Objection to blood transfusions for religious or cultural reasons.

Advantages of Minimally Invasive Surgery

Minimally invasive surgery avoids the need for the heart-lung machine and its associated risks (page 23). A blood transfusion is less likely, so it is a viable option for patients who refuse blood products. You will avoid the large incision in the middle of your chest, and your smaller incisions are less likely to become infected (although they may be more painful). Patients who have had MIDCAB have a shorter stay in the intensive care unit and usually go home within 3 days. So why doesn't everyone have MIDCAB?

Disadvantages of Minimally Invasive Surgery

MIDCAB is suitable for only a very specific group of patients (see More Detail box on page 69), and is most successful for treating blockages in the left coronary artery. The long-term success of this procedure is not known, because it has not been around very long and many surgeons report that short-term success is unsatisfactory. The grafts may not be as good technically due to the fact that the surgeon cannot see the site as clearly (although surgeons who are experienced with this procedure will assure you otherwise). There is also the risk that you will have an incomplete surgery if the surgeon cannot reach all the blockages or that you will be switched to traditional bypass surgery to complete the job. Finally, the incisions may be more painful than a breastbone incision. For all these reasons, MIDCAB is a fairly uncommon procedure.

What Happens Next?

Just as in traditional bypass surgery, you will be monitored carefully after your off-pump or minimally invasive procedure. Chapter 8 tells you what to expect as you recover in the cardiovascular intensive care unit.

Chapter 8

when it's all over

What Happens in this Chapter

- Wires and tubes in the intensive care unit
- Waking up
- Transfer to the ward
- Managing pain and moving around
- Care of your wound
- Medical complications
- Leaving hospital

Once you leave surgery, you will spend about 24 hours in the intensive care unit before being transferred to the ward. The aim of your care team is to help you feel normal as soon as possible, without any complications. When all your body systems are stable and you can move around easily, you will be allowed to go home. Most patients leave hospital about 5 days after their bypass surgery.

Day 1 – The Intensive Care Unit (ICU)

Most ICUs are large, open rooms in which each bed is surrounded by equipment and separated from another by a curtain. When you arrive in the ICU, a specialized medical team will take over from your surgical team to keep a careful eye on you around the clock. Many of the wires and tubes you had in the operating room will come with you into the ICU and be linked up to monitoring equipment beside your bed. A special nurse and an ICU physician will also check your heart and lungs the old-fashioned way—with a stethoscope.

In addition, a respiratory therapist will attach you to a ventilator to help you breathe and an X-ray technician will take a picture of your chest to confirm that tubes are in place and your lungs have expanded properly. Your nurse or physician will attach your temporary pacemaker wires (page 63) to a pacemaker box in case it is needed. The team will also check your blood pressure and send blood samples to the lab to measure your blood hemoglobin, clotting times, and cardiac enzymes. This will tell them whether you need a **blood transfusion** (hemoglobin) or an adjustment to your **blood-thinning drugs** (clotting times), and how your heart reacted to surgery (enzymes). These tests will be repeated over the next few days to check your progress. The fluid draining from your chest and your urine output will also be recorded regularly.

> "I kind of marveled at how busy the ICU seemed. There was a lot of coming and going—a lot of activity."
>
> **Ian Gillespie**

You may be very cold and shivery when you arrive at the ICU. It is not uncommon for body temperature to fall as low as 25°C during bypass surgery. The heart-lung machine should warm your body to 35°C before it is disconnected, but you may still arrive at the ICU in need of warming blankets to get you back to a normal 37°C.

The blood that is draining from your chest tubes may be returned to you using an **autotransfusion**

device. You may also require a blood transfusion at this time, either of donated blood or your own pre-donated blood (see page 32 for a detailed discussion of blood-transfusion options).

In the ICU…
It's All About You

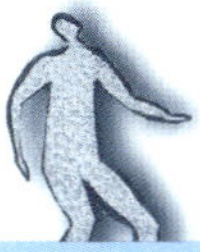

[MORE DETAIL]

The intensive care unit can make you (and your family) feel helpless and afraid, but knowledge is power. Here's how all those wires, tubes, and other equipment are speeding your recovery.

What Is It?	**What Does It Do?**
Arterial line – a thin tube in your arm	Checks your blood pressure and blood chemistry
Intravenous (IV) line – another thin tube in your arm, neck, or both	An easy way to administer medicines and fluids
Drainage tube – a tube in your chest	Drains fluids from your surgical site
ECG – soft pads on your chest	Measures your heart rhythm
Pulse oximeter – a clip on your finger	Measures oxygen in your blood
Pulmonary artery catheter – a tube in your neck to your heart	Checks the pressures in your heart
Ventilator – a breathing tube	Helps you breathe
Pacemaker wires – fine wires protruding through the skin of your chest	Can be connected to a pacemaker if your heartbeat becomes slow or irregular
Chest X-ray	Confirms your tubes are in the right place and checks on your lungs
Warming blanket (optional)	Increases your body temperature after you leave the cold operating room

Family and Friends

Once your surgery is over, your surgeon will want to talk to a member of your family or another supporter. If friends or family need to leave the waiting area during your surgery, they should tell a member of staff where they are going. If they leave a phone number, remind them to keep the phone line open at all times until you are out of surgery and the surgeon has been in touch.

Waking Up

When you wake up, be prepared. The ICU is like nowhere else you've ever been. You will gradually regain consciousness to bright lights, beeping and humming equipment, ringing telephones, conversations around you, and constant activity. Busy, caring people will be coming and going. You'll lose all track of time. You'll hear, "Your surgery is over and you are fine" and feel far from fine. But be assured: you're being looked after, you're doing well, and you're on your way to recovery.

"I remember them taking the breathing tube out. That wasn't a big deal."

Mel Isen

Ventilation and Breathing

When you first wake up you may become aware of a tube in your windpipe. This is connected to a ventilator machine that is helping you breathe. You will also notice that the ventilator is inflating and deflating your chest and that you are not able to speak. Many people don't like the idea of the ventilator tube, but be assured that as you become fully awake and start to breathe independently, the tube will be removed if all your body's vital signs (temperature, blood tests, chest tube drainage) look normal. You will then be given an oxygen mask or nasal prongs instead.

Before removing the breathing tube, your nurse or respiratory therapist may need to clear your throat with a suction tube. Although this can be uncomfortable—some people describe a sensation of pressure and suffocation—it only takes a matter of moments and will help you breathe properly afterward.

Chest Tubes

The tubes in your chest are used to drain the extra fluid or blood from the site of your surgery so that it does not pool around the heart or lungs. The tubes will be removed as soon as the flow of fluid becomes a trickle—usually by the time you leave the ICU.

Urinary Catheter

This tube is placed in your bladder to allow urine drainage and measure the quantity. This is usually removed in the ward, after you leave the ICU. Some older men with prostate enlargement may have some irritation afterward or difficulty voiding. This usually settles down in a day or so, but if the problem persists a urologist will be called in to assist you.

[SELF-HELP]

Memory lapse

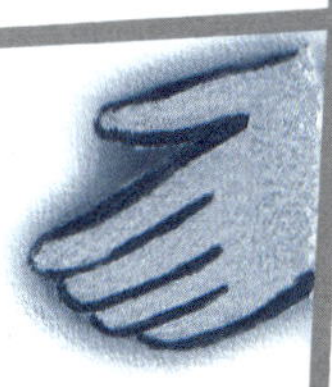

It is not unusual to have no recall of the ICU experience. This may be due to the combined effects of the general anesthetic and pain relief and the short stay.

Removal of Your Tubes and Lines

Many of the lines and tubes attached to you in the ICU will gradually be removed as you recover and they are no longer needed. You will probably go to the ward with just an IV line, the pacemaker wires and the urinary catheter. Removal of your chest tubes may be uncomfortable, but the rest of the lines usually come out with little or no discomfort. Think positive: each time a tube is removed, it is a sign that you are making progress.

Days 2 To 5—The Ward

You will leave the ICU as soon as you no longer need continuous monitoring, one-to-one nursing, or intravenous drugs. This is usually around 12 to 24 hours after surgery. On the ward, little by little, you will be encouraged to regain your independence.

You will now return to the care of your surgical team. This means that you may see your surgeon every day. Unlike the ICU, on the ward you will no longer have your own nurse. Instead, there may be one nurse to four to six patients. Some people worry that this change means their problems may go unnoticed. This is unlikely, but if you are concerned, discuss it with your nurse, who will always be close at hand.

Your first full day on the ward will be busy. Your urinary catheter will probably be removed, along with your chest tubes if they are still in place. You will be encouraged to get out of bed and gradually start to breathe room air instead of wearing your oxygen mask or nasal prongs. You will move from clear fluids to solid food, depending on how you're feeling.

"It was 3 days before I even put my feet near the floor. I had to have somebody on both sides of me the first time I did get out of bed just to walk the length of the bed. I was pretty weak. But I came home in 7 days."

Jim Morning

How Will You Feel on the Ward?

Everyone is different, so it is difficult to predict exactly how quickly you will improve after your surgery. However, be assured that by days 3 or 4 most people report that their pain has been reduced to discomfort only.

You may feel tingling from your chest incision, or a grabbing, tight pressure, especially when turning in bed and moving around. There may be a short, stabbing pain when you cough (see Self Help box on page 79). Using your leg muscles to move in and out of bed instead of your arms and upper body will help reduce discomfort.

If you have a leg incision, it will feel sore when you first get up to walk. Any stiffness should go away as you exercise. Taking pain medication before you exercise and wearing loose clothing to prevent rubbing should help.

As well as pain from surgical sites, many people report discomfort from their shoulder, neck, and back muscles, and difficulty sleeping. Some women experience a dull, heavy breast discomfort. Most of these symptoms are normal and will improve with time. However, any sharp, piercing pain may mean something needs attention and you should tell your nurse about it immediately.

Tests and Measurements

While you are on the ward, your medical team will give you a detailed daily examination to check for anything that needs to be adjusted. You should report anything that is bothering you. Your blood pressure, heartbeat, and the amount of oxygen in your blood will be measured, and your nurse will also watch for fever, pain, and difficulty breathing. You may also need to leave the ward for repeated X-rays or **cardiac ultrasound**.

Pain Management

There are many options for pain management and your nurses will make sure that you are comfortable. During the first few hours after surgery the pain medication you were given in the operating room should continue to work.

If you need to have the chest tubes in for more than a few hours, you may be fitted with a self-controlled pain-relief device called **patient-controlled analgesia (PCA)** that allows you to give yourself small amounts of medication whenever you need it. Simply press the button and a preset dose of pain relief (usually morphine) is infused directly into your vein through your IV line. It takes about 5 minutes to give relief, so press the button as soon as your pain starts to increase or about 5 minutes before doing something painful (e.g., coughing exercises). If it doesn't seem to work, wait a few minutes, then press the button again. This can be repeated until you are comfortable. PCA is controlled, so you cannot receive too large a dose. If you are not getting pain relief after several uses, tell your nurse.

[KEY POINT]

Don't be afraid you'll become addicted to your pain relief. Studies have shown that people who take morphine for pain have little trouble stopping, although pain relief may cause side effects such as drowsiness and nausea. Tell your nurse about side effects, but don't reduce your medication.

By the second day of surgery, your pain relief will probably be in the form of tablets or suppositories, such as Tylenol No.3 or Percocet (see page 133).

Pain management works best when the blood level of the medication remains constant, so ask for pain medication frequently (every 3 to 4 hours as needed). This will stop your pain from building up, allowing you to move or exercise more easily and sleep more comfortably. There are a lot of myths about taking pain medications, such as a drug addiction (see Key Point box) or the belief that experiencing pain is a sign of strength. Be assured that regular dosing is better for you and will prevent you from taking larger doses to get your pain under control. If you find that despite taking medications you are still experiencing a lot of discomfort, tell your nurse or physician. There are several combinations that they can use to make you more comfortable.

One of the side effects of some pain medications is constipation, and this is made worse by your lack of activity immediately after surgery. To keep things moving along you'll be given a stool softener each day and don't forget to drink plenty of water (except if your fluids are being restricted). Eating fruit, vegetables, and fiber cereals will also help. Your family can bring in healthy meals prepared at home if you don't like hospital food.

Breathing

Your physiotherapist or nurse will encourage you to breathe deeply and cough to re-expand your lungs (see Self Help box). He or she may also want you to use a machine called the **incentive spirometer**, a "lung exerciser" that gives you feedback on how deep your breaths really are.

[SELF-HELP]

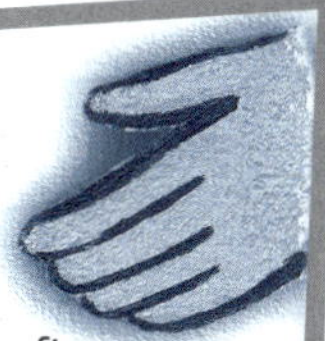

Have a Good Cough

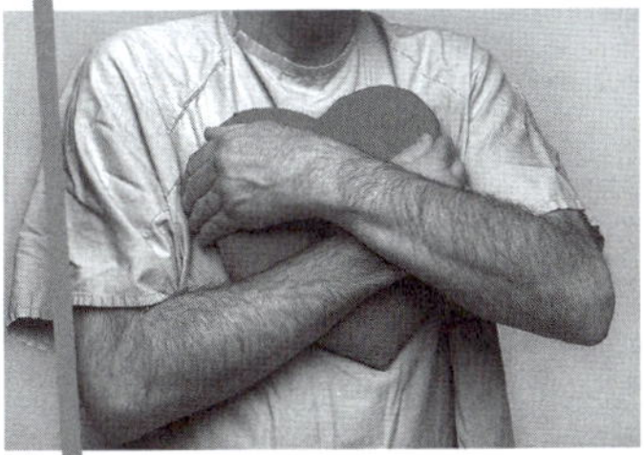

Coughing is good for you after bypass surgery—even though it may not feel like it—because it removes fluids from your lungs. Holding a pillow to your chest as you cough and taking pain medications on time will help reduce your discomfort.

Wound Care

Your incision and graft site will be cleaned regularly with **saline** (salt water) and covered with a dry, sterile dressing for the first 24 hours after surgery. The dressing will then be removed. The incision may feel tight, sore, or numb, and the surrounding skin may look bruised or slightly red. This will improve with time. You may also notice some clear, pinkish fluid draining from your chest incision; this isn't unusual.

Antibiotics

To reduce the chances of an infection in your surgical site (or anywhere else), you will probably be given antibiotics as a precaution. The type of antibiotic varies from hospital to hospital. You should tell your doctor before surgery if you are allergic to antibiotics. For more on antibiotics, see page 128.

Water Balance

You may gain up to 5 percent of your total body weight in extra fluid during surgery due to the water that was added to your blood in the heart-lung machine. You should lose this fluid during the first 36 to 48 hours as your kidneys get to work through a natural process called **diuresis**. This may take longer in people with a weakened heart or kidneys and may require drugs called **diuretics** to speed up the process. Your nurse will check how you are doing via your urinary catheter, which you will wear for up to 48 hours after surgery. Your catheter will be removed some time on the second or third day after surgery, if all is well.

> "The other symptom I had, which I noticed was very common, was hiccups...one of the things that really helped me was flat ginger ale."
>
> **Mel Isen**

Pacemaker Wires

Your temporary pacemaker wires (see page 63) will be removed about 4 days after surgery. Some patients feel nothing; others describe the process as a strange pulling sensation. You will need to rest for about 30 minutes afterward.

Activity

From the day after surgery, you will be expected to gradually increase your activity to prevent blood clots forming in your veins (**deep vein thrombosis**). Your physiotherapist will work out an exercise plan with you for 5 to 20 minutes of activity several times a day. Starting with leg-pumping exercises while you are still in bed, you will be encouraged to walk greater and greater distances around the ward until, within a few days, you will be climbing stairs. Move slowly, with relaxed deep breathing, and stop if you feel pain. Wear good walking shoes with rubber soles and firm support.

When Things Get Complicated

Some people have complications—unwanted medical symptoms or illnesses—after surgery (see More Detail box on page 82). Many of the precautions that we have already described, such as antibiotics or exercise, are aimed at reducing the chances of complications, but you should be aware of them in case they happen to you.

Atrial fibrillation, or an irregular heartbeat, is very common and happens in up to one-third of patients. It usually starts on the second or third day after surgery. This is why your heart rhythm is monitored. You may be unaware of it, or you may experience an alarming, rapid heartbeat. Your care team will treat it with medication or an external pacemaker using your pacer wires (page 63). It will probably go away by the time you leave the hospital.

Heart attack can happen in up to 1 in 20 patients, but is becoming less common as surgical techniques improve. It is usually mild and well-tolerated, and is treated with medication. It is more likely to occur in people with unstable angina.

Some people, especially those who had kidney disease before surgery, can suffer partial or complete **kidney failure**. This often improves by itself. It is rare in people with healthy kidneys (1 in 100 cases) and occurs more often in older patients, those with diabetes or poor heart function, and long or complicated operations. In the hospital, it may be treated with kidney dialysis.

Forewarned Is Forearmed

[MORE DETAIL]

This is a list of the complications (unwanted medical events) that your medical team will be watching for in hospital and treating, if necessary.

What?	**How Common Is it?** (percentage of patients)
Irregular heartbeat (atrial fibrillation)	20 to 30%
Post-operative confusion	1 to 25% (very variable)
High blood pressure	20 to 30%
Kidney failure (people with pre-existing kidney problems)	16%
Kidney failure (people without pre-existing kidney problems)	1%
Heart attack	3 to 5%
Fluid build-up around the heart or lungs severe enough to need treatment	3 to 4%
Severe stomach problems (ulcers or gastritis)	0.5 to 3%
Significant wound infection	Less than 1%
Any infection	4 to 6%

About one-third of patients suffer from **post-operative confusion** for a few hours or days. They may be disorientated, speak strangely, and act oddly or aggressively. This can be very disturbing for families if they are not prepared. It is probably due to the anesthesics, other medications, and lack of sleep associated with surgery. It is more common after long, complicated operations and in older patients. It is also more common in those who drink a lot of alcohol, so patients and families should be open and honest when asked about alcohol consumption before the operation. A small number of patients may need sedation to prevent injury to themselves or staff.

Depression, or the "post-op blues," is common on the second or third day after surgery, but usually clears up by itself. Family and friends can help by being supportive and optimistic.

Stroke can happen during or after bypass surgery (see page 25). Strokes are rare in younger patients and are more likely to occur in patients over 75.

The last thing many patients expect after heart surgery is stomach problems, but **peptic ulcers** and stomach pain (**gastritis**) happen in about 1 in 100 bypass patients. To prevent this, your physician may put you on medications to protect your stomach until you start to eat normally.

Your chest tubes are designed to drain excess fluid from your surgery site, but occasionally problems arise due to fluid building up where it shouldn't. A condition called **cardiac tamponade**—in which blood builds up around the heart and makes it hard for it to beat—sometimes requires further surgery or insertion of a small drainage tube. It happens in the first 1 to 7 days and is usually treated before you are aware of it. About 4 in 100 people need an extra drainage tube to treat fluid around the lungs (**pleural effusion**).

Infection of your surgical sites is always a hazard after surgery, although your team will be doing all they can to prevent it. If your incision becomes infected, the site will be sore and tender and you may develop a fever. Antibiotics and good wound care usually solve the problem. If the infection is inside your chest, you may need further surgery.

Going Home

You should be ready to leave the hospital in 4 to 7 days. Most people go home on day 5. You may have some of your stitches and staples taken out before you leave and the rest will be removed in 1 to 2 weeks. You will be given prescriptions for all the medicines you will need and instructions on taking them. Your care team will also give you plenty of counseling (and written instructions) on everything from wound care to follow-up appointments. You should receive contact information for your nearest **cardiac rehabilitation program** (page 97) and be encouraged to attend. You will be given a 24-hour emergency number to call if you have any problems.

What Happens Next?

Once you get home, there is plenty you can do to speed your recovery. Your anxious family may want to restrict your activity, but staying active is one of the most important things you can do to improve the health of your heart. Take things step by step and listen to your body as you walk the road to recovery. The next chapter outlines where you go from here.

Chapter 9

recovering at home

What Happens in this Chapter

- Medical support after discharge
- Sleeping, driving, sex, exercise, food
- Getting back on your feet
- Incision care
- Dealing with medications
- Managing pain and discomfort
- Emotional changes
- Cardiac rehabilitation
- Returning to work

Heart surgery, like any major surgery, places a great deal of stress on your body. At first you may feel as though you will never get better. Try not to be discouraged. Many people have trod this road before you and things will improve over the next few weeks. By gradually increasing your activity, joining a cardiac rehabilitation program later on, and staying involved with friends and family, life will eventually return to normal.

Medical Care After Your Discharge

It is normal to feel uncertain or have questions when you leave the hospital – some patients even fear going home. But it is important to remember that your medical support does not end just because you have been discharged. You will be given a 24-hour telephone number before you leave the hospital in case you have any problems or concerns when you first get home. A nurse or nurse's assistant may also come to your home, if you arrange this, to help you take care of your wounds and with daily activities, such as climbing the stairs.

Although timelines for follow-up appointments vary from place to place, typically you will have an appointment with your family doctor 1 week after your discharge. You will see your cardiologist within one month, and up to 3 months after you leave the hospital, you will have an appointment with your cardiac surgeon.

[SELF-HELP]

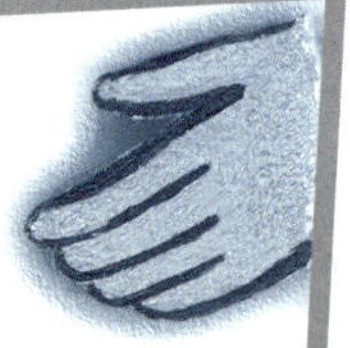

When to Call Your Doctor

Call your doctor if you experience:

- Fever greater than 38.5° C or 101° F
- Excessive drainage that is red or full of pus
- Redness, swelling, or pain from your incisions
- Swelling in your legs or hands and a weight gain of around 6 pounds in 1 week
- Severe pain in your chest, back, or shoulders, especially if it increases with a deep breath
- Your heart beating very fast or "skipping a beat" when you are resting

Sleeping

Some people have trouble sleeping for several weeks after bypass surgery. This is perfectly normal. For the first few days or weeks you may find it works best to sleep when you need to and not worry about insomnia. If you are determined to get back into a nighttime routine, these tips may help:

- Avoid caffeine and alcohol
- Go to bed every night at the same time
- Try a nighttime ritual that helped you sleep in the past, such as reading or sipping a hot drink
- Take your pain medication or sleep medication before going to bed
- If turning in bed is difficult, try sitting up first and then turning

Driving

Because some of the medications you are taking can cause drowsiness, you shouldn't drive for 4 to 6 weeks after surgery. Also, if you stop suddenly while driving, contact between the steering

[SELF-HELP]

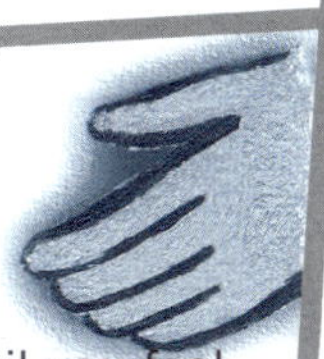

Driving Tips

- Start by driving in local areas and avoid highways until you feel much better.
- Wearing your seat belt will not harm your incision.
- Use a towel or small pillow to prevent rubbing or irritation on your incision.
- You may still have some chest or neck stiffness when you turn.

wheel and your breastbone can disturb the healing process. You may, however, ride in a car for the first few weeks of your recovery. If you need to take a long journey, be sure to stop at least once every hour and walk around for about 5 minutes to get your blood circulating.

You should contact your insurance company to see if they have any specific guidelines regarding driving after major surgery.

Eating and Drinking

Your appetite will take a few weeks to return to normal after surgery. Some people say that their taste for food is gone or that foods taste abnormal, for instance, metallic, very sweet, or salty. Unless your doctor or dietitian tells you otherwise, eat a well-balanced, nutritious diet until your appetite returns.

As you get stronger and your appetite returns to normal, it is important that you make the switch to a heart-healthy diet. In essence, you should try to eat much more fiber, fruit, and vegetables and reduce all fats, especially saturated fats. Food is an important part of life and any dramatic change can be difficult, so get some help (see Chapter 10).

Drink 6 to 8 glasses of water a day unless your doctor tells you something different. Some people may need to restrict their fluids. Try to limit caffeinated drinks such as coffee, tea, or cola to 2 or 3 servings each day, or switch to a decaffeinated brand. Alcohol may be unwise for certain people (see page 104), but be guided by your physician.

Sex

Many people find that they are not very interested in sex after heart surgery. Don't worry—this is not permanent. There are no rules about when you can or should resume your sex life. The time will be right when you and your partner are ready. Try building up gradually to your normal level of sexual activity by starting with something simple, such as hugging, kissing, or touching.

Sex, like any exercise, increases the heart rate and blood pressure, but it is not as hard on your heart as you may think—about equivalent to climbing two flights of stairs. If you experience a rapid heartbeat or have difficulty breathing for 20 or 30 minutes after intercourse, have angina pain, or feel very tired the next day, consider slowing the pace down a bit. In time, the partner who has had a heart attack or heart surgery is usually able to resume the same activity level as before (if not more so).

[SELF-HELP]

Sex after Surgery

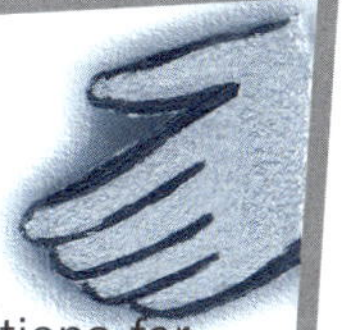

The American Heart Association gives the following suggestions for lovemaking after a heart attack. These tips are also useful for people who have had heart surgery.

- Choose a time when you are rested, relaxed, and free from stress brought on by the day's responsibilities.
- Wait 1 to 3 hours after a meal to allow it to digest.
- Select a familiar, quiet setting where you are unlikely to be interrupted.
- Take medicine before sexual activity, if prescribed by your doctor.
- Find a position that does not put pressure on your breastbone, such as on the back (for men) or side by side.
- Take it easy. Allow adequate time for foreplay, both to get your heart going gradually and to recapture some intimacy after spending time apart.

Physical Activity

Week 1

For the first week to 10 days, gradually increase your level of activity from what it was in the hospital. Remember to:

- Rest as much as possible for the first day or two when you arrive home.
- Continue with the breathing, arm, and leg exercises you learned in the hospital.
- Take several short walks with rest periods in between rather than one long walk.
- Gradually increase the length of your walk if you can.
- Avoid extremes of temperature (too hot or too cold).
- Try not to feel frustrated – routine activities, such as showering, dressing, eating, and resting will take longer and may consume the entire day.

"I found company very tiring. People mean to be kind and come and see you, but it can be very tiring. You just feel like you're at your wits end."

Marie M.

After the first couple of days, begin to climb stairs slowly. Hold onto the handrail and take one step at a time. It's best to lead with your good leg first and rest every fourth step for about 30 seconds when you are going up the stairs. When you are going down the stairs, lead with your bad leg first. Because climbing stairs takes a lot of energy, do not go up or down the stairs more than once or twice a day for the first 2 weeks.

Week 2

By the second week, you can start increasing your activity level by trying to lift and carry light objects (less than 10 lbs or 5 kg) for short distances. An example of 10 pounds is a loaded grocery bag.

You can also increase the distance you walk. Start by doing one block per day and increase that distance gradually to four blocks (two blocks each way). You can avoid temperature extremes by walking during the middle of the day in the winter, and during the evening or early morning in the summer. Try indoor activities, such as using a stationary exercise bike, during bad weather.

> "The first two weeks were pretty bad. Probably about the third week I was able to move around with a lot more mobility."
>
> **Ian Gillespie**

[SELF-HELP]

Recovery Do's and Don'ts

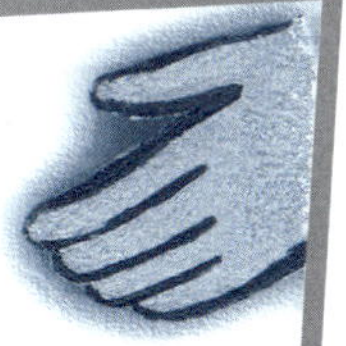

DON'T...

- Open stuck windows
- Push, pull, or reach with your arms
- Resume household chores too soon (women tend to do this)

DO...

- Take part in short social gatherings
- Some light housework, such as setting the table, dusting, or washing dishes
- Gradually resume your sexual activities
- Start to go up and down the stairs the way you did before surgery instead of taking one step at a time
- Get plenty of sleep every night
- Join a cardiac rehabilitation program (page 97)

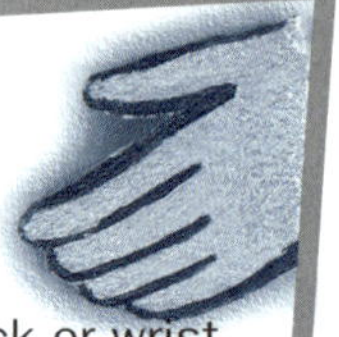

What's My Heart Rate?

To work out your heart rate, first find your pulse in your neck or wrist. Count the pulses for exactly 6 seconds and add a zero.

E.g., 7 pulses in 6 seconds = heart rate of 70

Always take your pulse before, during, and immediately after you finish exercising (see Self Help box). Your heart rate during exercise should be at least 10 beats per minute higher than your resting heart rate, but no higher than 120. Your pulse should return to its resting rate within 15 minutes of finishing your workout. If you feel pain when you exercise, stop, rest, and consult your doctor. The easiest way to figure out if you're doing too much physical activity is to take the talk test—you should be able to talk while exercising, or you are working too hard. If you can sing while you are exercising, you need to work a bit harder.

"All of a sudden, one day I was up in the kitchen and I didn't realize I'd walked up the stairs by myself. Now that was a plus!"

Cora Billing

Weeks 4 and 5

During the fourth and fifth weeks, continue your breathing, arm, and leg exercises. You should gradually increase your walks to at least 30 minutes per day and you can start doing chores, such as light yard work, washing the car, or preparing meals. At this point, you can discuss returning to work with your cardiologist. If a hospital in your area offers cardiac rehabilitation, this might be the time for you to begin.

Weeks 6 to 8

After 6 to 8 weeks, your breastbone should be healed and you can gradually resume all the activities that you did before your surgery. Continue to exercise. If you are not sure what exercise to do, discuss it with your doctor, nurse, or physiotherapist. With your doctor's permission, you may also return to work full time.

Incision Care

Caring for your incisions is an important part of your recovery. Start by gently washing your wounds every day with a clean washcloth, mild soap, and warm water while you are in the shower. Rinse your wounds well and pat them dry with a clean towel. Avoid putting dry-skin ointments or creams on the incision. Look for any new drainage, redness, or swelling, and be aware of signs of infection, such as heat at the site of the incisions or feeling feverish. Some tricks to help ease the discomfort of your healing wounds are to wear loose clothing, take your pain medications, and hug your chest with a pillow when you cough.

If your sutures are not dissolvable, or if you have any remaining staples, you may need to go to your family doctor 1 week after discharge to have them removed.

Chest Wound

It will take 1 to 2 months for your chest wound to heal completely. Your chest bone will be tender, so try not to bump or scratch it. Women may find wearing a bra while sleeping is helpful, to avoid pull on the incision line. Some women use front-closing bras because they don't have to reach around to close them, while others prefer bras that close in the back because they are less irritating to their chest scar. If you find that a button-down shirt irritates your scar, try taping a gauze bandage or thin sanitary pad to the inside of it, or wear a T-shirt made of soft fabric instead.

Graft Wound

If your graft was taken from your arm or your lower leg, you may have some swelling or bruising around the incision. Elevating your arm or leg for 15 to 20 minutes will help to reduce the swelling, especially after exercising. You can also wear below-the-knee supportive stockings that will help prevent fluid from accumulating. Finally, if your incision was in your leg, you should avoid crossing your legs while sitting.

Medications

While having bypass surgery will improve your health, it does not mean that you will be able to stop taking medication. Some of your medications may be different after you have your surgery and you will be given any new prescriptions on the day that you are discharged from the hospital. Take only those medications prescribed by your surgeon until you see your own doctor. If you have any questions, contact your doctor or pharmacist.

[SELF-HELP]

Tips for Taking Medications

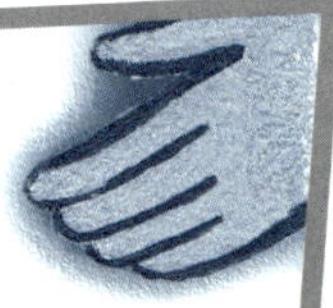

- Review your medications with your doctors during follow-up visits.
- Try to take your medications at the same time every day.
- Check with your doctor or pharmacist before buying non-prescription medications.
- Keep your medications in your carry-on luggage when traveling.
- Use a pill organizer if you are on many medications.

For more information on medications, see Chapter 12.

Management of pain and discomfort

Each patient experiences pain differently. After heart surgery, you may feel discomfort in your chest for a number of weeks. You can reduce your pain by taking your pain medication before any activity.

You may also feel discomfort due to constipation as a result of your pain medication, reduced activity levels, or iron supplements. Whatever you do, don't strain to try and force a bowel movement. You can relieve your constipation by:

- Eating foods high in fiber, such as fruit and whole grain breads and cereals
- Drinking 6 to 8 glasses of liquids per day
- Anything you usually do to help move your bowels
- Drinking milk of magnesia in the correct doses
- Inserting a Dulcolax suppository in your rectum if milk of magnesia doesn't work
- Using a fleet enema if Dulcolax doesn't work.

You can get the medications mentioned above without a prescription at the drug store.

Emotional Changes

The feeling of relief you may have after your operation can sometimes be followed by more negative feelings, such as mood swings, depression, irritability, and a lack of energy. These feelings are a normal part of the recovery process and can be caused by anesthesia, medications, loss of sleep, or the stress of

"The physical recovery will take longer than you anticipate. But I think some of the biggest challenges are going to be psychological and emotional."

Ian Gillespie

[SELF-HELP]

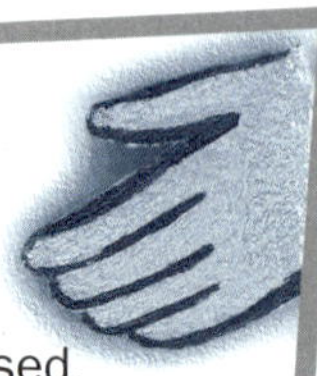

Dealing with Depression

- Each day, no matter how you feel, get washed and dressed, and prepare yourself for some activity.
- Talk out your concerns with close family and friends.
- Join a cardiac rehabilitation program (page 97).
- Tell your doctor if your negative feelings don't go away after a couple of weeks.

surgery. The support of friends and family, returning to work, and becoming involved in other activities will usually help you feel better. If you feel bad for more than a week or two, you should talk to your doctor who can help you decide whether professional counseling or medication may be beneficial.

Peer Support

While family and friends can offer valuable encouragement, some patients find that support from people who have also experienced bypass surgery is more helpful. Some cities have peer support groups that meet to talk about members' experiences with life after bypass. Your local hospital should be able to put you in touch with these groups, and some groups are listed in Resources (see page 152).

Cardiac Rehabilitation

Cardiac rehabilitation ("cardiac rehab") is a support program aimed at returning heart patients to an active, healthy life. Most programs begin around 3 months after surgery and require a referral by your family doctor or cardiologist. The hospital will give you all the information you need about cardiac rehab before you go home. Joining a cardiac rehab program is one of the best things you can do for your heart—and yourself.

Cardiac rehabilitation usually involves weekly or monthly classes, spread out over several months. The first, intensive part of the program involves a multidisciplinary team of physicians, exercise physiologists, nurses, occupational therapists, social workers, physical educators, lab technologists, and support staff. They will work out where you are now, and where you need to get to, and design an exercise and lifestyle program tailored to your own needs.

Studies have shown that patients who attend cardiac rehab have better recoveries than those who don't. The most important feature of cardiac rehab is the support that you will receive. Many people find exercise, lifestyle changes, and recovery from surgery difficult, both physically and emotionally, and even family members can't always say or do just the right things. The team at cardiac rehab, and the other patients in the program, understand what you are going through and can give you exactly the right kind of advice and support for a healthy and happy recovery.

Returning to Work

Getting back to work is a realistic goal after heart surgery and can be a psychological boost—a sign that things are "getting back to normal."

> "The other thing that really made a difference was the program at the rehab center ... That was fabulous. First of all you're with a group of people who have had similar problems. Secondly, the people there were able to monitor me. I think a lot of it is psychological. They told me how much I could walk and I felt comfortable with that and they checked me out to make sure that that was okay. It was just great to go there every week. People should have their doctor make the referral right from the hospital because it does take a while."
>
> **Mel Isen**

Patients generally wait until after their 4-week check up with their cardiologist before deciding when to return to work. The time it will take you to return to work will depend on the kind of work you do, although you will probably get permission to go back about 6 weeks after surgery. Until then, you can keep an eye on things at work via email or phone, if necessary. If your job is stressful or physically demanding, you may have to wait longer to go back (up to 3 months) than someone whose job is less strenuous. Many people switch to a less strenuous job or start back part-time at first.

What Happens Next?

When you are feeling stronger and have fully recovered from your surgery, you may want to consider making lifestyle changes. Your bypass operation has not cured your heart disease and to stop it from getting worse, you need to take stock of how you live. The next chapter shows you how to get back in control of your heart disease—and your life.

Chapter 10

how you can help yourself

What Happens in this Chapter

- Lifestyle shifts that can transform your future
- Changing your diet—the simple and easy way
- Exercising your way forward
- Supplements and herbal medicines
- Massage, visualization, acupuncture, relaxation
- The science of complementary therapies

You are the most important part of your care team. It may not feel like it when you are undergoing surgery and in other people's hands, but be assured that you can make all the difference to the success of your bypass surgery. A long-term commitment to exercise, dietary changes, and quitting smoking can transform your future health. Learning a technique for positive thinking and relaxation before your surgery will give you the power to control your stress and discomfort and speed your recovery.

Healing Your (Whole) Self

In this chapter we will look at ways in which you can improve your heart health through exercise and diet. We will also explore techniques such as visualization and relaxation and other complementary therapies that you can use to help you prepare for your bypass procedure and take control of your life afterward.

Most of the therapies mentioned use a holistic approach to your health. The word "holistic" comes from the Greek word *holos* meaning "whole." Holistic health care involves treating the whole person and not just one isolated body part or one risk factor. When you are considering what you can do to help yourself, think of healing your whole self and not just your heart.

[SELF-HELP]

Help Yourself to a Healthy Heart

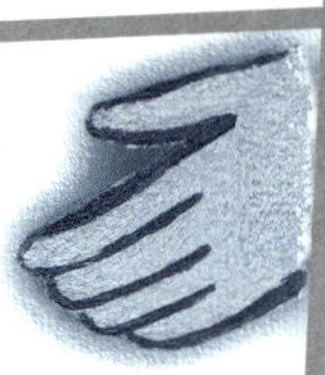

The "big four" (M.E.D.S.)

- **M**anage stress
- **E**xercise
- **D**iet
- **S**moking (stop)

Some people also find these approaches helpful:

- Vitamins and supplements
- Herbal medicines
- Visualization and relaxation techniques
- Massage, therapeutic touch, and acupuncture

Healthy Lifestyle and Heart Disease

The old adage "you are what you eat" holds a great deal of truth, particularly when it comes to heart disease. Heart disease is a disease of over-fed countries. It is important to take a step back, take a good look at your diet, and plan out what improvements you should make.

Many studies have shown that healthy eating can stop your heart disease from getting worse. However, it must be a long-term commitment. Improving your diet for only a short period of time will make no difference to the health of your heart because atherosclerosis—the artery-hardening process that causes heart disease—is a chronic (long-term), not an acute (short-term), disease.

Changing the eating habits of a lifetime can be hard, especially if you aren't very confident in the kitchen. Most hospitals can refer you to a cardiac rehabilitation program or dietitian who will give you plenty of encouragement and practical advice. There are also lots of heart-healthy cookbooks to help you (see page 154).

What Is a "Heart Healthy" Diet?

Healthy eating involves eating a well-balanced diet containing foods from all the main food groups. No one food group alone can provide you with all the necessary nutrients needed to maintain health.

"I quit smoking and turned to fruit."

Cora Billing

Fruit and Vegetables

There is plenty of evidence to show that a diet rich in fruit and vegetables helps to protect against and, potentially, reverse cardiovascular disease. Fresh fruit and vegetables are high in nutrients and fiber and low in calories. The exact reasons why they protect against heart disease is unknown. Part of the reason may be that a diet rich in high-fiber foods is likely to contain less saturated fat, a major cause of heart disease (and obesity, another risk factor for heart disease). It is also likely that there are active ingredients within fresh fruit and vegetables that help the body fight disease, including heart disease. The active ingredients are unknown, so beware of expensive supplements in health food shops that claim to be full of them. Try to eat at least five servings of fruit and vegetables each day and, if possible, eat local organic produce and what is currently in season because these may be fresher and contain more nutrients.

Fiber

Most of us don't eat enough fiber, so it makes sense to boost this important part of your diet. This should help to reduce your cholesterol level and, because fiber fills you up without adding calories, it will also help to reduce your calorie intake and lower your body weight. You can get more fiber by incorporating plenty of fresh fruits and vegetables, as well as whole grains, nuts, and cereals (oatmeal, wheat germ, whole oats, etc.) into your diet.

Fats

When you're trying to choose heart-healthy food it can get pretty confusing trying to sort out what you're meant to be doing about those fats. Dietitians now keep the advice simple: reduce your fat intake overall and *especially reduce saturated fats*. The easiest rule of thumb for managing this is to avoid products high in animal fats —all those hamburgers and hot dogs. The reason for this is that most animal fat is saturated fat.

If you wish to eat dairy produce, try to stick with the lower-fat or non-fat products. These would include skim or 1 to 2 percent fat milks, low-fat yogurt, and low-fat cheeses. Try using polyunsaturated or monounsaturated margarines for spreading on baked potatoes, bread, or other baked goods, and olive or canola oils for dressings, sauces, and frying.

How Low Do You Go?

There is a scientific debate raging, particularly in the U.S., over whether very low-fat diets (containing around 10 percent of calories from fat) can actually reverse heart disease. Some studies appear to support this idea, while others seem to show that once you get down to a certain point (about 25 percent), there is no further benefit gained from reducing fat. The debate will no doubt continue to get more interesting, but in the meantime, the advice in Canada is to aim for about 30 percent of calories from fats (many people find that hard enough), and reduce saturated fats and trans fats.

"It always helps when you have a supportive family."

Marie McVety

Protein Sources

Use a variety of protein sources such as fish, soy products, lean meat, poultry, and legumes. If you do eat meat, stick to lean cuts and small portions. There is good evidence to show that eating at least one portion of oily fish per week (such as mackerel and sardines) has a heart-protective role in coronary heart disease (see page 112, "Omega-3 fatty acids").

Beans, nuts, and legumes are great sources of protein and thus can be used as an alternative to fatty meats, as can soy products. Nuts and seeds also contain polyunsaturated fats (the "good" fats).

[KEY POINT]

Diets are hard, so let's keep the rules simple. Eat much more fiber, fruit, and vegetables and significantly reduce your total fat intake, especially saturated fats.

Salt

It is a good idea for all heart patients to limit their salt intake. Avoid prepared foods, processed foods, and take-out-type foods, which are generally high in salt. The current recommendation is less than 3 grams of salt per day—about half a teaspoon. Ask your doctor before using a salt substitute.

Alcohol

Alcohol can be a pleasant part of social occasions, but it can also be harmful for people with heart disease. Alcohol is also extremely high in calories and thus contributes to weight gain, so moderation is the key. Avoid alcohol completely while you are taking prescription pain medication or if you have raised triglyceride levels in your blood. Some heart medications should not be combined with alcohol; it is best to check with your pharmacist if you are unsure. If your doctor allows alcohol, limit your intake to 1 ounce of liquor, 1 beer, or 4 ounces of wine per day.

Check Your Weight

It's hard, we know it is, but if you have heart disease, achieving and maintaining a healthy body weight is essential. Weight gain is associated with an increased risk of coronary artery disease and stroke. If you lose weight you may also reduce your blood pressure. The more gradual your weight loss, the greater the chance that the weight will stay off. "Crash diets" are an unsafe way to diet and, in the majority of cases, the weight will be regained. A consultation with a registered dietitian can help you work out what your ideal

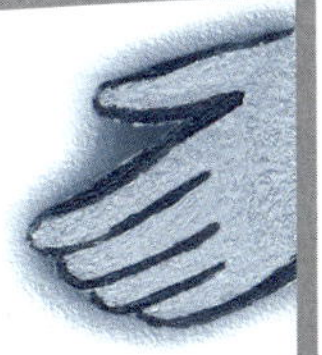

Help Yourself to a Healthy Diet

The following are some tips to help you eat your way to health:

- Take a heart-healthy cooking course. It will be fun, you'll meet other people in the same position as you, and you'll learn how food can be delicious as well as healthy.
- Load up on fruit, vegetables, and fiber at every meal. That way you'll have less room for fatty foods.
- Try to use broths instead of gravy.
- If you eat meat, each portion should be no bigger than the palm of your hand.
- Remove the saltshaker from the table. Use other flavorings such as fruit juice, herbs, and spices.
- Watch those "low-fat" bakery and dessert items. They are often very high in sugar, so you'll put on weight—which is also bad for your heart.
- Be aware of hidden saturated fats. Not all food labels list the saturated fat content. Be particularly suspicious of baked goods and pre-prepared meals.
- Avoid deep-fried foods. They are usually high in saturated fat or they may have a lot of **trans fats** (hydrogenated vegetable oils), the worst kind of fat for your heart.

weight should be and help you set goals to achieve it. Keeping to the healthy diet guidelines above may be all that is needed to shed the extra pounds.

Check Your Blood Pressure

High blood pressure is the "silent killer" because it usually has no symptoms but makes your heart disease worse. If you have heart disease, you will almost certainly be taking blood-pressure-lowering medication, but you can further reduce your blood pressure with lifestyle modifications, in particular, losing some weight and reducing your salt intake.

Check Your Cholesterol

The most important thing you can do to lower your cholesterol, in addition to taking your cholesterol-lowering medicine, is to reduce the amount of saturated fat that you eat. There is also some evidence that soluble fiber, found in foods such as oatmeal, can lower blood-cholesterol levels.

[SELF-HELP]

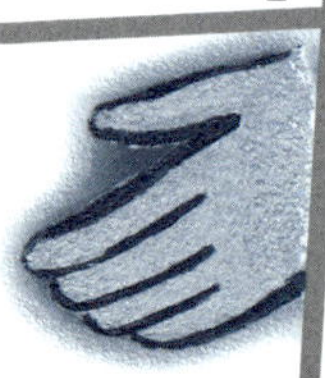

Use the diary pages of this book to record and track your lifestyle goals. You can also use them to keep track of all your medications, including complementary medications.

Cigarette Smoking

There is overwhelming evidence that smoking is, without question, disastrous for the health of your heart. The good news is that it is never too late to stop. Your risk of a heart attack or death falls rapidly once you stop smoking—by as much as 40 percent, according to one study. There is advice and support available to help you give it up. Talk to your GP, cardiologist, or cardiac rehabilitation program.

[KEY POINT]

It's never too late to give up smoking.

Exercise

We all know about it, we've all done it (some of us still do it), not many of us do enough of it, and we all know how good it is for us.

Exercise is essential. There are no alternatives to it and you alone are responsible for doing it, since no one can do it for you. Exercise can play a huge role in your recovery and long-term well-being. It can help you lose weight, it may lower your blood pressure, and may even stimulate new blood vessels to grow in your heart. Choose a sensible exercise program that suits you. The general guidelines in Canada recommend that adults should do 30 minutes of moderate exercise at least 5 days of the week. Moderate activities are cycling, fast walking, swimming, or heavy-duty housework.

"With exercise I became normotensive for years. I learned to walk at a proper pace so as not to stress myself. I now walk a minimum of 6 hours a week. If I walk more I don't get credit for it, but if I walk less I have to make up for it next week."

T. Hofmann

Get a Helping Hand

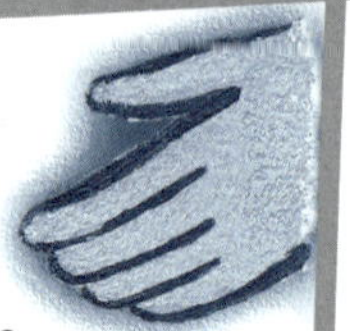

We strongly recommend that you enrol in a cardiac rehabilitation program, which will give you specific targets to aim for, general support, help, and advice based on your individual needs (see page 97)

Stress Management

Our lives today contain enormous amounts of stress. Stress is the body's "fight or flight" response with nowhere to go, so the burden that stress places upon the body is huge. It acts as a silent and slow-acting body debilitator—almost like a disease in itself when it is left unattended. It can be years before we realize just how much stress we are under. It can take years, again, to actually recognize that we need to do something about it. Even if we try to ignore stress, our bodies are extraordinarily clever at giving us warning signs that we are overdoing things. It is essential that you learn to recognize these signs and do something about them.

"Stuff doesn't bother me the same as it did before. If something went wrong, I'd get really upset and kind of worked up about it, but now it doesn't bother me the same. After the operation I thought, 'What am I worried about here?'"

Jim Morning

Following are a few ideas that you might like to consider to control or manage your stress. See also Relaxation, Meditation, and Massage (pages 114–116).

Go for a Walk

You may not feel like it at the time, but once you get outside a walk can do wonders for clearing your head and lowering your blood pressure.

Deep Breathe

Sit down somewhere quiet (even if it means sitting in the washroom), and inhale and exhale slowly and deeply. As you breathe out, try to imagine all your anger or frustrations being blown out with your breath. Say to yourself, "I do not need this stress, my health is more important." Repeat this to yourself a few times before you go back to what you were doing.

[KEY POINT]

Stress is potentially dangerous for heart health. However, there are many simple ways to deal with it. The key is to find a method of stress management that you feel comfortable with, to provide relief for your heart (and your head!).

Try to Avoid Arguments and Conflict

Avoiding a fight may be easier said than done, but nothing raises the blood pressure more effectively than a heated argument. Once again, ask yourself if the issue that is making you angry or frustrated is more important than your health. Is it possible to wait a few minutes or hours when all those involved in the conflict have calmed down? Perhaps then the issue at hand can be discussed more rationally and quietly.

Get Plenty of Sleep

Lack of sleep can only add to the stresses of the day. You can improve your chances of a good night's rest by

- not having caffeine after 4pm
- going to bed at the same time every night
- trying to sleep only when you're tired
- having a comfortable mattress
- buying some earplugs if your partner snores

Find a Hobby

Outdoor hobbies such as gardening are particularly helpful for stress. They can re-focus your mind and stop you from thinking about things that make you feel stressed.

Take Your Watch Off

Our lives are ruled by time. How many times in a day do you look at a clock or a watch? Find a day when you have nothing planned, take your watch off, and spend the day doing what you want, according to how you feel. Eat when you are hungry, rest when you feel tired, and fill in the rest of the time your way. You will be amazed at how re-energizing this can be.

Vitamins and Supplements

If you eat a well balanced diet (see above), it should provide you with all the essential nutrients and vitamins you need to achieve optimum health. You should consider vitamins and supplements only if you are not able to maintain a well-balanced diet.

If you have ever walked into a store selling vitamins and dietary supplements you will know that it can be overwhelming and confusing. If you are considering taking a supplement, seek out a professional such as a dietitian, qualified nutritionist, or naturopathic doctor who can recommend what you need to best complement your diet.

Multivitamins

Studies have shown that high doses of multivitamins can be unhealthy for heart disease patients. If you are considering multivitamins, consult a qualified professional.

Vitamins C and E (the antioxidant vitamins)

Despite many scientific studies, there is still no clear-cut evidence that vitamin C and E supplements make any difference one way or another to heart disease patients. It seems that vitamin E at a dose of 100 to 400IU daily, combined with a diet high in fruits and vegetables and plenty of exercise, *may* be beneficial in heart disease patients. For vitamin C, there is still no overwhelming evidence that it is beneficial as a treatment for heart disease when taken as a supplement. In fact, the Los Angeles Atherosclerosis Study recently showed that high doses of vitamin C (850mg to 5,000 mg/day) may make matters worse. This study found that artery disease progressed *faster* in patients taking these high doses of vitamin C, than it did in patients who did not take vitamin C supplements.

So why did some studies show a benefit and others did not? One possible explanation of why the vitamin supplements were ineffective in some of the studies is that the patients were sticking to a healthy diet and receiving adequate vitamin C and E anyway, so the supplements were unnecessary.

[KEY POINT]

It is *essential* to inform all people involved in your care what supplements and medicines you are taking to avoid the risk of dangerous drug interactions. Physicians need to know about all non-prescription medicines and supplements; complementary therapists need to know about prescription drugs.

Folic Acid, B6, and B12

There has been a lot of interest in these supplements as a treatment for heart disease because deficiencies in these vitamins can cause high blood levels of an amino acid, linked to cardiovascular disease, called **homocysteine**. However, there is not, as yet, evidence to show that these supplements prevent or reverse atherosclerosis. A better choice might be simply to eat more fruit and fresh vegetables.

Co-enzyme Q10

Co-enzyme Q10 is a naturally occurring enzyme found within the body tissues, particularly in the heart, liver, and pancreas. To date, there have been no substantial studies on humans to prove its benefit for treating heart disease when given as a supplement (despite what the Internet may tell you).

Omega-3 Fatty Acids

Omega-3 fatty acids have been shown to have a protective role in coronary heart disease. To obtain your omega-3s without supplements, eat at least one fatty-fish meal per week or incorporate flax seeds, flaxseed oil, hemp seed oil, canola oil, and nuts into your diet.

Herbs

Herbs have been used as medicines since the beginning of humankind, and many of today's prescription medicines are based on natural substances found in herbs. Although there are numerous herbs advocated for use in heart disease, clinical studies have only been carried out on a few. Hawthorn has the most overwhelming evidence that it works.

Hawthorn

In large, well-designed clinical studies similar to those carried out on prescription drugs, hawthorn has been shown to increase blood flow to the coronary arteries, strengthen the heartbeat, and decrease blood pressure. It also has antioxidant properties and minimal side effects. Hawthorn is widely used throughout Europe as a medicine for the heart, often in combination with conventional drugs. However, hawthorn can affect the blood levels of other drugs, such as digitalis, glycosides, beta-blockers, and other blood-pressure-lowering drugs.

KEY POINT

Because of the blood-thinning effect of garlic, you should stop taking it (either raw or in capsules) at least 10 days prior to your surgery or you may be more susceptible to bleeding. If you are thinking of starting garlic capsules and you are already taking other blood-thinning medications, talk to your physician.

Garlic

There is good scientific evidence that garlic can protect your heart. One study, published in the *Journal of the Royal College of Physicians and Surgeons of London* in 1994, showed that eating 1/2 to 1 clove of garlic per day can reduce cholesterol levels by as much as 12 percent. Other reputable studies have shown that it has a blood-thinning effect, by reducing the stickiness of platelets (see Glossary), and can reduce the stiffness of the main blood vessel of the body, the aorta, in elderly people.

Ginko Biloba

Ginko is not as well-researched as hawthorn and garlic, but there are a few studies that show it increases blow flow and is an effective treatment for some circulatory diseases. A recent review of all studies, published in the *American Journal of Medicine* in 2000, concluded that ginko is particularly beneficial for treating artery disease in the blood vessels of the legs.

Other Herbs for Heart Disease

Other herbs used to treat cardiovascular disease for which there is scientific evidence include Terminalia arjuna, a traditional Ayurverdic herb used for heart conditions since the sixth century BCE, and tumeric. A recent study published in the *International Journal of Cardiolology* showed that Terminalia arjuna has benefits for patients with heart failure. Tumeric appears to have anti-platelet, cholesterol-lowering, and antioxidant properties.

The following herbs have been traditionally used to lower blood pressure, although there are no reputable scientific studies to either prove or disprove their effectiveness: olive leaves, cramp bark, yarrow, dandelion leaves, lime flowers, and mistletoe.

Safety Note

It must be *strongly* advised that if you are considering exploring the use of herbs to assist you with your health you consult an experienced herbalist or naturopathic doctor. Herbs and prescription drugs can interact, with serious side effects.

Other Complementary Therapies

Relaxation

It is widely recognized within the medical profession that people who learn to relax can control symptoms and, in some cases, even reduce blood pressure or pain. Relaxation can be achieved in a number of ways, including meditation, yoga, deep breathing, a nice hot bath, or simply imagining yourself lying on a hot, sunny beach. The trick is finding ways to relax in your current anxious state. Many cardiac rehabilitation programs now teach relaxation techniques as an integral part of recovery and it is useful to learn a relaxation technique to prepare for your surgery. There are numerous tapes and books on relaxation, so check out your local bookstore.

Meditation

Sit in a quiet place, focus on your breathing, and find a word or phrase that you can say over and over again to yourself. For example, you might try phrases that rid you of negative feeling towards other people and help you to accept personal differences. Letting go of such destructive feelings will give you more energy to focus on your own health and well-being. You might also consider a meditation program such as Tai Chi or yoga.

Visualization

This is a form of meditation that involves using mental imagery to bring about the changes that you wish for. The idea—a visual version of "positive thinking," which may explain its apparent success in some people—is to believe that the more clearly you can see your desired future, the more chances there are of it becoming true. Many people find that visualization works well for surgery. You could visualize the surgery itself and welcome it in a positive way, seeing it as a means to an end, a necessary part of the healing process. It works best if you divide the images into the different stages of surgery, such as, going to the hospital, preparing for surgery, the surgery itself, returning to the ICU, and returning to your regular life. You can buy tapes to help you with visualization. Although they are not designed specifically for bypass surgery, they will give you tips and techniques to help establish a positive mindset about your surgery.

Acupuncture

Acupuncture has been in use for over 3,500 years in China and involves inserting fine needles into the skin and underlying tissues. Acupuncture practitioners consider acupuncture to work by

The Science of Complementary Therapies

[MORE DETAIL]

Complementary therapies for heart disease are, *generally speaking*, not as widely researched as conventional drugs or surgeries and the studies that do exist are often not up to the standard of conventional drug trials. This means that we don't always know about side effects or how people with different diseases might be affected, so be cautious. A therapy isn't safe just because it's "natural" (the natural world contains some of our most powerful poisons). There are, however, a surprising number of good studies and the science of complementary therapies always makes for fascinating reading. See Resources at the back of this book.

stimulating the "vital force" or *qi* (pronounced chee)—the spiritual, mental, emotional, and physical aspects of a person. Although science has neither proven nor disproven that acupuncture works this way, what we do know is that it can relieve angina and anginal-type symptoms in some people.

Massage

Massage is the art of using the hands to stimulate the skin and muscles to bring about a feeling of comfort and to promote healing. The Bible, the Qur'an, and the Ayur-Veda all mention the use of massage. There are many forms of massage, including Swedish, shiatsu, aromatherapy, reflexology, and neuromuscular. It can be a very positive experience and is the perfect way to reduce stress.

Chelation Therapy—Does It Work?

Chelation therapy has been in use for approximately 40 years in North America for many different chronic illnesses. Heart disease patients generally receive chelation therapy intravenously (into a blood vessel). The theory is that chelation agents improve circulation by removing undesirable elements such as calcium and toxic metals from the blood, thus helping to reduce disease in the walls of blood vessels.

Intravenous chelation therapy in heart disease is extremely expensive and there are *no* reliable clinical trials proving that it works. If you are considering chelation therapy you should think about it carefully, given the potential for adverse side effects, the expense, and the lack of any documented benefit.

> "You have to work at it. Exercising, losing weight, changing diet, it's hard. A positive attitude is the best thing."
>
> **Robert (Bobby) Frew**

What Happens Next?

If you have heart disease, no drug or surgery will work by itself. Likewise, no complementary therapy should be considered an "alternative" therapy, that is, a replacement for medical intervention. A combination approach—medical therapy, diet, exercise, other complementary approaches—is going to give you the best chance of slowing your heart disease and returning you to health. Be sure to always tell your doctor about any complementary treatment that you decide to undertake. Likewise, be sure to tell any complementary practitioner about your surgery.

You are now well equipped to take full control of your heart's health. In the next chapter we look at the long-term results of bypass surgery and how you can decide whether the procedure worked for you.

Chapter 11

has my bypass surgery worked?

What Happens in this Chapter

- How you might feel right away
- What you might expect over the next 12 months
- The long-term picture

In most people, coronary artery bypass surgery relieves angina symptoms, improves quality of life and increases life expectancy. Expect to take a few months getting back to normal, though, as your body recovers from your operation. The length of your recovery will depend on many factors, including your health before your surgery. If all goes well, you should feel better than you did before your surgery within 3 to 6 months.

You and your physician will decide whether your surgery was successful mainly by how you feel—are your angina and quality of life better than before your surgery? If required, your physician can also carry out the same tests that were used to diagnose your heart disease. To track your progress, you will probably see your cardiologist 2 to 4 weeks after you get home, and your cardiac surgeon up to 3 months later.

Some time during the first year after your surgery you will probably have a repeat exercise test to see how your heart is doing.

Immediate Results

Don't expect to feel better right away. In the first few days after surgery you should be free of your angina pain, but any benefit may be overshadowed by tiredness and the discomfort of your incisions. Some people mistake this discomfort for angina. You should improve rapidly, however, and by the time you go home you will feel much better.

Figure 11–1. Your New Bypass Graft

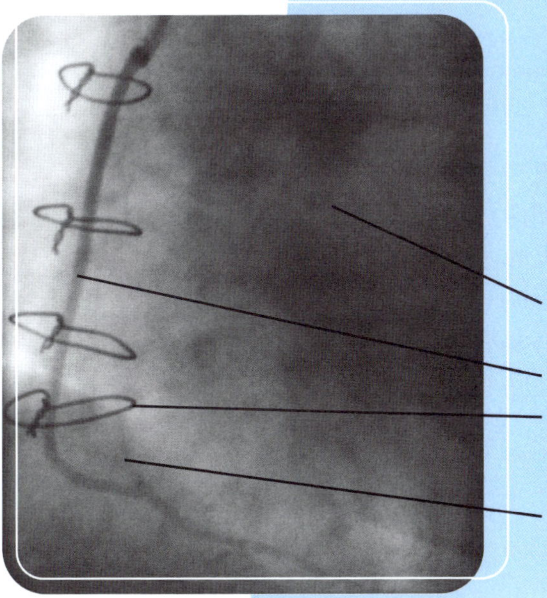

This X-ray picture (angiogram) shows a new bypass graft in place. Blood can be clearly seen flowing through the graft.

The Recovery Period

Hopefully, you will be free of angina symptoms for many years after your surgery. Results vary widely from patient to patient, but studies show that less than 3 percent of patients develop angina within a year of bypass surgery. If you do experience angina symptoms in the first year after surgery, you need to inform your doctor and develop a plan for managing them.

So what about quality of life? Many people say that they feel tired all the time after bypass surgery. Be assured that this is temporary and that you should regain your strength within a month to 6 weeks. Do not be discouraged if you seem to be making no progress or have bad days. Be patient and take it one day at a time. The tiredness will go as you gradually get back to your normal activities. Studies show that most people return to normal activities within 3 to 6 months after surgery and by 1 year most people feel as good or better than they expected (see More Detail box).

> "I had to just accept that it had to be done and I wanted to live to see my grandchildren grow up."
>
> **Marie McVety**

A number of important factors will affect how quickly you recover from your surgery. The most important is your previous medical history. You may experience a longer, or less successful, recovery if you have had a recent heart attack, unstable angina, or heart failure,or if you still have an irregular heartbeat, heart-valve problems, obesity, and other medical issues such as diabetes, stroke, and problems with your circulation, breathing, or kidneys. Emergency bypass surgery may also mean a longer recovery than planned surgery.

Older patients (over 65) can do very well after bypass surgery. Although studies show that older patients are more likely to have medical complications that prolong their hospital stay, the good

Recovery Timeline

[MORE DETAIL]

In the authors' experience, most patients feel better than before their surgery within 3 to 6 months. Your own recovery may be faster or slower than this, as shown by many studies that have looked at recovery in bypass patients. A timeline from one such study is shown below.

First 2 months	Difficulties sleeping, eating, doing normal activities
4 months	Most patients can climb stairs, walk, garden, drive Half of patients can do heavy work
6 months	Resumption of normal activities Most feel better than before surgery 1 in 8 still feel worse
1 year	Lives back to normal for most patients 3 out of 4 say recovery is as good as or better than expected

news is that once they are out of the hospital, their quality of life improves just as dramatically as that of younger people.

Women tend to take longer to recover than men, partly because women tend to come into the hospital for bypass surgery less fit and sicker than men, and have greater domestic responsibilities once they get home. On the other hand, studies show that women have fewer mental health problems after bypass surgery and tend to view it as a normal event of aging, while men see it as a major life-threatening event.

It is important to realize that recovering after bypass surgery is an active, not a passive, process. A positive attitude to the changes in your life can make a huge difference to how quickly you get back to normal. One study found that patients who were tense and anxious at 4 weeks after surgery were less likely to have returned to normal activities at 8 weeks.

Joining a **cardiac rehabilitation program** (page 97) is one of the best ways to recover—both mentally and physically—from your surgery. You will receive the support you need and a recovery program designed especially for you.

Partial Revascularization

> "We're the fortunate ones. We do go through a lot, but in the end it's worth it."
>
> **Mel Isen**

During traditional bypass surgery, most people have bypasses successfully placed in all their diseased blood vessels (**complete revascularization**). However, sometimes it is not possible for the surgeon to bypass all the blocked vessels, for instance because some vessels are too small. This is called **partial revascularization**. Such "incomplete" results are also found after angioplasty and are common after off-pump bypass surgery (see page 68). If this is the case, your surgeon should explain what happened and warn you that you may still get angina symptoms that require medical treatment.

The Long-Term Picture

Traditional bypass surgery has good long-term results. Ten years after surgery:

- Up to 95 percent of arterial grafts are still functioning
- Up to 90 percent of patients are still alive
- Around 90 percent of patients have not had a repeat bypass operation
- 92 percent of patients have not had angioplasty

To prolong the survival of your grafts (and your heart) it's important to realize that bypass surgery has not "cured" your heart disease. If you do nothing, your heart disease will continue to get worse and you may need another procedure in the future. This is more likely if you continue to smoke, do not control your blood cholesterol through diet and medication, and don't exercise. Bypass surgery at a young age or a partial revascularization also make another bypass more likely in the future.

What Happens Next?

Your long-term health, including the need for a repeat procedure in the future, depends on what you do next. Your heart is in your hands. Read Chapter 10 for some ways in which you can slow the progression of your heart disease and help yourself to a healthier future.

Chapter 12

medications

What Happens in this Chapter

- Medication guidelines
- Medications to treat heart disease
- Medications used before surgery
- General anesthetics
- Medications used after surgery

Now, more than ever, you are the most important part of your own care team. You should be clear on why you are taking the medications you have been given, how to take them, and what they are for. It is also useful to know about possible side effects so that you will be able to recognize them and tell your physician if they occur. This chapter is a quick guide to medications you may be given before, during, and after your surgery.

Pre-Hospital Medications

There are hundreds of drugs to treat diseases of the heart and blood vessels (**cardiovascular drugs**), and the likelihood is that you are taking one or more before your surgery.

Cardiovascular drugs have three main purposes:

- To prevent or reduce the number of angina attacks that you have (beta-blockers, calcium channel blockers, ACE inhibitors, and nitrates)
- To treat angina attacks if and when they occur (nitrates)
- To prevent the disease in your blood vessels becoming worse (anti-hypertensives, anti-platelet agents, anticoagulants, and lipid-lowering drugs)

The full list of medications your physician will prescribe depends on many factors, including whether you have had a heart attack, have high blood pressure, or have some other medical problem.

Your physician will probably continue (or add on) some of these drugs after your surgery, particularly the drugs that prevent your heart disease from getting worse. These are needed because bypass surgery does not "cure" heart disease, so you will need to keep taking these drugs after your surgery—sometimes for many years.

Cardiovascular drugs that you may be given are divided into the following groups. Specific drug names are in the table on pages 132 to 133.

Nitrates

Nitrates, such as nitroglycerin, are used to both prevent and treat angina attacks. They have been in use for more than a century. Nitrates widen blood vessels, thereby increasing blood supply to the tissues (including the heart muscle) and reducing the amount of work the heart needs to do.

Beta-Blockers

These drugs reduce blood pressure, heart rate, and the strength of the heart's contraction. As a result, the heart needs less oxygen. **Beta-blockers** have been used for more than 20 years.

[SELF-HELP]

Help Yourself to the Right Medications

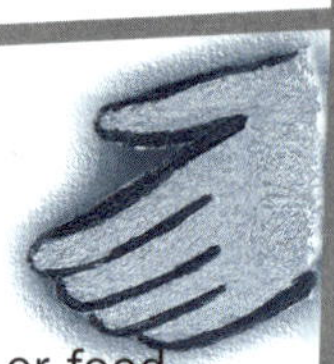

- Tell your doctor or nurse about any medication or food allergies.
- Always tell health professionals about other medications that you are taking, such as complementary therapies, drugstore medicines, or supplements.
- Never stop a medication or cut the dose without first consulting your physician—even if you start to feel better.
- If you miss a dose, don't take double: just take the next dose as usual.
- Never take someone else's medications.
- Ask your doctor or pharmacist about possible side effects and report any unusual effects or reactions.
- Reorder medications before they run out to give your pharmacist time to order.
- Always carry a list of the medications that you are taking, and a note of what they are for. You may wish to use the diary pages at the back of this book.

Calcium Channel Blockers

Also called **calcium antagonists** or **CCBs**, these drugs relax the muscles around blood vessels, thus widening arteries and increasing the blood flow and oxygen delivery to the heart muscle. They have been available since the 1980s. They are used for treating high blood pressure and angina, as well as reducing the chances of a radial artery graft going into spasm.

Angiotensin-Converting Enzyme (ACE) Inhibitors

ACE inhibitors are a relatively new class of drugs, mainly used to treat high blood pressure and heart failure. However, they have also been shown to stop angina from getting worse by having a beneficial effect on the lining of blood vessels, to prevent heart attacks, and to strengthen the heart muscle after a heart attack.

Anti-Platelet Agents

Once a blood vessel is narrowed by atherosclerosis, a blood clot can form on the blockage, causing severe angina or a heart attack. **Anti-platelet agents** reduce the tendency of blood platelets to form blood clots. There are a number of different ones with different uses, depending on how potent they are. ASA (Aspirin) is the best-known example of an anti-platelet agent that can be taken every day. If you cannot tolerate Aspirin, you may be offered clopidogrel (Plavix) instead.

Anticoagulants

Anticoagulants also prevent blood from clotting, through a different mechanism from the anti-platelet agents. You may be prescribed an anticoagulant such as warfarin (Coumadin) as preventative medicine, or you may be given one (such as heparin) if you need it during your hospital stay.

Lipid-Lowering Drugs

Lipid-lowering drugs reduce the level of cholesterol and other fats in the blood. This helps to prevent your heart disease getting worse by slowing down further narrowing of your coronary arteries.

Other Blood-Pressure-Lowering Drugs

Beta-blockers, calcium channel blockers, and ACE inhibitors (see above) all reduce blood pressure in addition to their benefits for angina. Other types of blood-pressure-lowering drugs, or **anti-hypertensives**, that you may be prescribed include the **diuretics** ("water pills") and **angiotensin-II receptor antagonists** (**ARBs**, for short).

Medications Before Surgery

Once you're in the hospital, you will be given two new types of medication before your surgery that each serve a different purpose.

Sedatives

You may be offered a **sedative** the night before your surgery and your anesthesiologist will give you one right before you're taken to the operating room. The purpose of a sedative is to help you feel more relaxed.

Antibiotics

You will also receive **antibiotics** intravenously (through a vein) before your operation to prevent infection during and after surgery. These antibiotics will be continued for 48 to 72 hours (depending on your hospital's protocol) after your operation. It's important to tell your doctor or nurse if you are allergic to penicillin, which is an antibiotic.

Medications During Surgery

Blood Thinner

A **blood thinner** such as **heparin** is needed when the heart-lung machine is used during surgery to allow the blood to flow freely over the artificial surfaces of the pumps and tubing. After your surgery is complete, the effects of heparin will be reversed using a drug called **protamine**. People with an allergy to fish or shellfish or diabetics taking protamine sulphate can experience problems with protamine at the end of surgery, so be sure to tell your doctor if any of these situations applies to you.

General Anesthetics

In the operating room, your anesthesiologist will give you medicines called **general anesthetics** that "put you to sleep." In fact, general anesthetics, which are given either through a vein (intravenously) or as a gas, do more than just put you to sleep. They also help with pain control, relax your muscles, and cause amnesia (loss of memory), allowing you to forget events immediately before and after your surgery.

The dosing for your anesthetics will be carefully calculated and adjusted based on your age, weight, past medical history, and the anticipated length of surgery. During surgery your anesthesiologist will make careful adjustments to your general anesthetics based on how you are responding. When you wake up you may experience side effects such as nausea, vomiting, disorientation, and headache, although this is relatively uncommon. If they happen to you, such side effects can be effectively treated and should go away within the first 24 hours after surgery.

General anesthetics have evolved greatly since they were first used. There is now a wide variety of different anesthetic drugs that provide a more controllable and safer kind of general anesthetic experience.

The stages of anesthesia can be broken down into **induction**, **maintenance**, **reversal**, and **recovery**.

Induction is the period in which you are "put to sleep," most commonly with an intravenous drug. The maintenance period is the time when the actual surgery takes place. Your anesthesiologist uses a combination of drugs to keep you asleep, relaxed, and pain free, either through your mask or intravenously. During reversal, special drugs are used to reverse the effects of anesthesia and wake you up. During the recovery phase you are monitored closely to make sure that all is well as you wake up.

After Your Surgery

Pain Control

Most people need powerful painkillers called **narcotics** (e.g., morphine) to be comfortable during their recovery. Pain control is an important part of your hospital stay, so it is covered in more detail in Chapter 8 (page 78).

Heart-Protective Drugs

After your surgery, you may be prescribed drugs to further improve the performance of your heart. **Digoxin**, a form of digitalis, improves the efficiency of the heart by making the heartbeat slower and stronger. Drugs called ACE inhibitors also improve the heart's pumping action in patients with poor heart function, as well as decreasing high blood pressure. ACE

[KEY POINT]

Any non-cardiac medications you were taking prior to surgery should be continued after your surgery unless you are instructed otherwise by your physician or nurse practitioner.

inhibitors may also have other long-term benefits for patients with coronary artery disease.

Anti-Arrhythmics

Anti-arrhythmics are drugs used to control your heart's rhythm. Surgery may make your heart muscle irritable, causing your heart to beat abnormally. These drugs will help prevent and control these abnormal rhythms. Beta-blockers and digoxin (see above) are used for this purpose.

Diuretics/Antihypertensives

Diuretics reduce blood pressure and **edema** (swelling) by increasing urine production. You may be given one or more diuretics after surgery to eliminate excess fluid and so decrease the workload on your heart. Your diuretics will probably be stopped by the time you are discharged to go home.

Stool Softeners/Laxatives

Stool softeners are prescribed after surgery to prevent constipation. A number of factors such as a low-fiber diet, immobilization, pain control drugs, and the surgery itself can cause constipation. Laxatives, which work by relaxing the bowel, will usually be prescribed for you for a period of 1 to 2 weeks once you are home.

Mineral Supplements

Potassium supplements are often prescribed in conjunction with diuretic therapy because diuretic medications can affect your salt and potassium levels. After surgery your physician may also prescribe an iron supplement to combat anemia due to losing blood during surgery. Iron supplements are generally continued for 4 to 6 weeks after surgery.

Medications and Potential Side Effects

Drugs	Common side effects
Nitrates e.g., isosorbide-5-mononitrate (Imdur, Ismo), isosorbide dinitrate (Cedocard, Coronex, Isordil), nitroglycerin (Minitran, Nitro-Dur, Nitrol, Nitrolingual, Nitrong, Nitrostat, Transderm-Nitro, Tridil)	dizziness, fainting, headache, low blood pressure, irregular heart rhythms, nausea, blurred vision, sweating
Beta-blockers e.g., acebutolol (Monitan,Sectral), atenolol (Tenormin), labetalol (Trandate), metoprolol (Betaloc, Lopresor), nadolol (Corgard), pindolol (Visken), propranolol (Inderal), timolol (Blocadren)	contraction of the throat muscles, tiredness, dizziness, low blood pressure, sleep disturbances, slow heart rate, cold hands and feet, diarrhea, constipation, nausea or vomiting, impotence, skin discoloration, fever
Calcium channel blockers e.g., amlodipine (Norvasc), diltiazem (Cardizem, Tiazac), felodipine (Renedil, Plendil), nicardipine (Cardene), nifedipine (Adalat), verapamil (Chronovera, Isoptin, Verelan)	headache, fast or slow heart rate, stomach upset, constipation, swollen tissues, dizziness, frequent need to urinate, palpitations, low blood pressure, flushing, tiredness, insomnia, muscle stiffness
ACE inhibitors e.g., benazepril (Lotensin), captopril (Capoten), cilazapril (Inhibace), enalapril (Vasotec), fosinopril (Monopril), lisinopril (Prinivil, Zestril), quinapril (Accupril), ramipril (Altace),	cough, low blood pressure, headache, dizziness, tiredness, nausea or vomiting, kidney problems, rash, altered sense of taste, swollen ankles, fever, joint pain
Anti-platelet agents e.g., abciximab (ReoPro), ASA (acetylsalicylic acid) (Aspirin), clopidogrel (Plavix), eptifibatide (Integrilin), ticlopidine (Ticlid), tirofiban (Aggrastat)	dizziness, chest or stomach pain, headache, rash, diarrhea, vomiting, flushing, swollen ankles, joint pain
Anticoagulants e.g., heparin (Hepalean), warfarin (Coumadin)	stomach pain, hair loss, blurred vision, rash, hives, itching, loss of appetite, diarrhea, skin discoloration, bruising
Lipid-lowering drugs e.g., atorvastatin (Lipitor), clofibrate (Atromid-S), cholestyramine (Questran), pravastatin (Pravachol), simvastatin (Zocor)	constipation, diarrhea, nausea, headache, stomach pain, indigestion, flatulence, muscle pain

Medications and Potential Side Effects

Drugs	Common side effects
Antibiotics e.g., cefazolin sodium (Ancef), vancomycin (Vancocin), linezolid (Zyvoxam)	diarrhea, oral thrush, nausea, vomiting, stomach cramps, skin rash
General Anesthetics e.g., midazolam (Versed), fentanyl (Sublimaze), nitrous oxide	nausea, vomiting, disorientation, headache for up to 24 hours
Narcotics (Pain Relievers) e.g., morphine, acetaminophen+codeine (Tylenol #3), acetaminophen+oxycodone (Percocet)	dizziness, lightheadedness, nausea, vomiting, dry mouth, constipation, drowsiness, disorientation, skin rash, sweating, low blood pressure, shallow breathing
Cardiac Glycosides e.g., digoxin (Lanoxin)	nausea, vomiting, headache, weakness, visual disturbances, slow heart rate, low blood pressure, flushing
Anti-Arrhythmics e.g., amiodarone (Cordarone), sotalol (Sotacor)	headache, fatigue, dizziness, impotence, muscle weakness, slow or fast heart rate, nausea, vomiting, altered taste, stomach upset, diarrhea, abdominal pain, hair loss, skin discoloration, blurred vision, low blood pressure, flushing
Diuretics e.g., amiloride (Midamor), bumetanide (Burinex), furosemide (Lasix), hydrochlorthiazide (Apo-Hydro, HydroDiuril)	fast or slow heart rate, electrolyte imbalance, low blood pressure, dry mouth, thirst, frequent urination, dizziness, weakness, nausea, vomiting, leg cramps, sweating, confusion
Stool Softeners e.g., bisacodyl (Dulcolax), docusate calcium, docusate sodium (Senokot-S)	RARELY – abdominal discomfort, nausea, diarrhea
Mineral Supplements e.g., ferrous sulphate (Fer-in-Sol), potassium chloride (K-Dur), potassium citrate (K-Lyte)	abdominal pain, nausea, dark stools, constipation, diarrhea

What About Side Effects?

All drugs have the potential to cause side effects. The goal is to avoid side affects or keep them to a minimum so that you don't notice them too much and they don't do any harm. Read the information that comes with your drugs or ask your pharmacist or physician about the possible side effects of your medication.

What Happens Next?

When you leave hospital with your new prescriptions, the next steps are up to you. Surprising as it may seem, many people with life-threatening conditions do not fill their prescriptions and, when they do, often fail to take the medication properly—or at all. By following your physician's instructions to the letter you are allowing your medicines to play their part in your recovery.

Chapter 13

future directions in cardiac surgery

What Happens in this Chapter

- Taking part in a clinical trial
- Some new advances in cardiac surgery

Cardiac surgery has taken great strides since the first heart bypass surgery was reported in 1967. Patients today can benefit from advances that continue to improve coronary artery bypass surgery and can help spur on these improvements by taking part in clinical trials. Future technologies include robotic techniques and therapies to encourage blood vessels to grow.

Clinical Trials and You

The key to all new medical advances is clinical research—research on real patients. The purpose of clinical research trials is to find out whether a particular medication, device, or technique is both effective and safe. Canadian hospitals are renowned worldwide for excellence in conducting clinical trials. If you are eligible to take part in any of these studies, you will be helping to test new treatments and playing a direct role in providing new options for heart disease patients in Canada.

Clinical trials may be sponsored by a pharmaceutical company, biotechnology company, or a government agency, but all trials must be officially approved by the hospital and independent ethics review boards before a study can begin. In most trials, neither patients nor researchers know until the end of the trial which patients are receiving the treatment itself or a **placebo** (non-active treatment). The advantage of this "double-blind" approach is that the results are non-biased. The disadvantage for patients is that they may not receive the new therapy—they may find themselves in the placebo group—or the new therapy may prove to be ineffective.

If you are interested in getting involved in a clinical research trial, your best bet is to ask your physician. The Internet is another good way to find out about clinical trials involving patients like you. When you are admitted to the hospital, you may be approached to participate in a clinical research trial; however, the decision is always yours.

New Advances in Cardiac Surgery

Robotic-Assisted Surgery

One active area of research is directed at making minimally invasive surgery easier. Instead of cutting open the breastbone, minimally invasive surgery involves going into the chest through small incisions between the ribs (see page 68), but there are limitations to this kind of surgery due to the restricted space inside the chest. A few research centers around the world are experimenting with robotic arms and cameras controlled by voice commands. These can provide the surgeon with video pictures that are 10 to 15 times larger than normal and allow for more dexterity inside a small working space—essentially providing the surgeon with an extra hand. However, although this technology is generating a lot of interest, it is likely to be limited to patients with disease in just one coronary artery (**single-vessel disease**).

Gene Therapy and Angiogenesis

A gene found in the lining of blood vessels may prove to be a useful adjunct to bypass surgery in the future, although research is still in the very early stages. This gene produces a protein called **vascular endothelial growth factor** (VEGF). When copies of the gene are injected into damaged heart muscle, heart cells secrete a substance that stimulates new blood vessels to grow. Gene therapy's role in the treatment of heart disease is currently being studied worldwide.

Transmyocardial Laser Revascularization

This technique, also known as **TMLR**, involves boring channels into the oxygen-starved heart muscle using a laser. This allows blood to seep into the heart muscle from the pumping chambers of the heart and may even stimulate the growth of the new blood vessels. TMLR has not been well studied, but it appears to give relief of angina symptoms for up to a year. It is generally reserved for patients who cannot have angioplasty or bypass surgery.

The Aortic Bypass Connector

For decades surgeons have used a needle and thread to sew new blood vessels into place during heart bypass surgery. Devices are currently in development that may allow surgeons to perform sutureless (no stitches) bypass surgery. One such device, the **aortic bypass connector**, uses a star-shaped rivet to clamp the vessel to the aorta in a matter of seconds (see Figure 13–1). Such techniques may be particularly useful in beating-heart surgery (see Chapter 7) where speed and dexterity are all-important, although the long-term safety and effectiveness of these devices are not yet known.

Figure 13–1. Symmetry™ Bypass System Aortic Connector

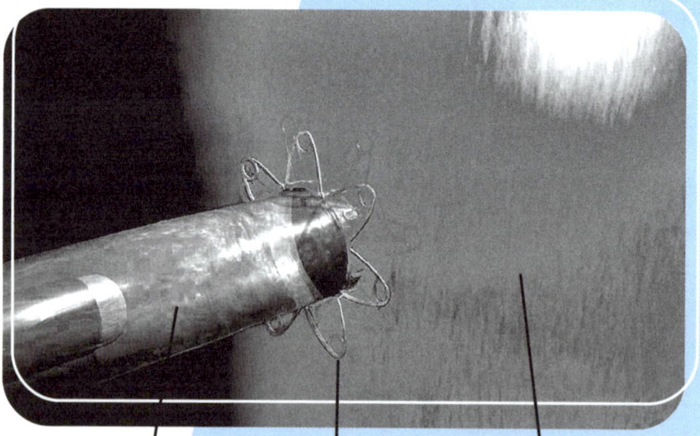

This device allows surgeons to attach bypass grafts with a star-shaped rivet instead of stitches.

Chapter 14

who's who of hospital staff

What Happens in this Chapter

- Hospital staff you will meet
- A brief description of their roles

When you go into the hospital, you will encounter a large number of staff. Generally speaking, the hospital staff will be friendly and approachable. If you are dealing with them directly, they should introduce themselves and explain their role in your care. Unfortunately, sometimes they are busy and unable to take the time to tell you how they can help you during your hospital stay.

To add to the confusion, many of the hospital staff, from porters to doctors, wear white coats or "scrubs" (loose pants and tops), making it hard to figure out who's who. In addition, within the title of "doctor" or "nurse" are a number of different roles, making it difficult to understand what each of these people do. For example, you may see a **fellow**, a **resident**, or a **staff physician**. All are doctors, but all have varying degrees of knowledge and ability, levels of training, and experience. Or, you may see a **ward nurse**, a **nurse practitioner**, or a **research nurse**. Again, all are registered nurses but each has a different role.

This chapter will give you a brief overview explaining who is who in the hospital and each person's role in your care.

[MORE DETAIL]

Medical Staff	**Nursing Staff**	**Ancillary/Support Staff**
Surgeon	Ward nurse	Nursing assistant
Staff cardiologist	Nurse practitioner	Ward clerk/receptionist
Anesthesiologist	Research nurse	ECG technician
Intensivist		Physiotherapist
Fellow		Occupational therapist
Resident		Dietitian
Intern		Social worker
Medical student		

Ward Clerk / Receptionist

Usually the first person you will meet upon your arrival to the ward. He or she is responsible for organizing the administration of the ward. Often his or her role extends beyond this, depending on experience level.

[KEY POINT]

Everybody you will meet in the hospital has a defined role. If you are not sure who somebody is, don't be afraid to ask.

Nursing Assistant

A person who has undergone training in patient care. However, his or her training is considerably shorter than that of a registered nurse. As a result, the nursing assistant is not permitted to perform certain procedures, such as administering drugs or inserting intravenous lines.

Ward Nurse

A registered nurse who works on the ward providing patient care. These nurses have a range of roles depending on seniority and experience. They are responsible for your well-being and safety during your stay on the ward.

Nurse Practitioner

A registered nurse who has completed a master's degree. He or she performs advanced physical examinations and takes patients' medical histories. The nurse practitioner is also responsible for coordination of patient care and patient education and works both independently and in collaboration with the health-care team in making rounds, ordering diagnostic tests, interpreting the results, and deciding on treatment.

Research Nurse

A qualified nurse who specializes in research. His or her role is to approach patients regarding possible participation in research studies and co-ordinate their involvement in the study.

ECG Technician

A person who is specifically trained to perform ECGs on patients. He or she may also assist in other areas that require heart monitoring, such as assisting with exercise-tolerance testing or Holter tape monitoring.

Medical Student

A person who is enrolled in medical school and training to become a doctor.

Intern

A person who has finished classroom medical-school training and is getting practical experience diagnosing and treating patients before specializing in a chosen area of medicine.

Resident

A doctor undergoing specialized training. He or she can specialize in a particular area, such as cardiac (heart) or thoracic (chest) surgery.

Fellow

Fully qualified doctors, specialized in a particular area of medicine or surgery, usually with a few years of experience. Many fellows come from other countries to spend up to 3 years gaining additional experience.

Staff Cardiologist

An experienced doctor who has undergone considerable training in cardiology and who is now in a position to make independent decisions regarding patient care and treatment. The staff cardiologist is responsible for your overall care on the ward and for the decisions made by more junior staff.

Cardiac Surgeon

A senior physician who specializes in cardiac surgery. He or she is responsible for evaluating your case before surgery, carrying out the operation itself at the head of the operating team, and making decisions about your care after your surgery.

Intensivist

This is a doctor who manages the medical care of patients in the intensive care areas of the hospital. He or she may be a resident or a fellow (see above) and is usually trained in anesthesia or internal medicine as well as intensive care. In the cardiac intensive care unit, an intensivist may be the only physician that you see.

Surgical Assistant

A doctor or nurse who assists the surgical team in the operating room, for instance by preparing vein grafts or closing incisions.

Anesthesiologist

A doctor who administers anesthesia to reduce or eliminate pain and put patients having surgery to sleep. The anesthesiologist's job includes medically evaluating patients before surgery, consulting with the surgical team, providing pain control, support of life during surgery, making decisions about blood conservation and transfusions, supervising care after surgery, and discharging patients from the recovery unit or intensive care unit.

Physiotherapist

Someone who is trained to work with patients to improve their physical function, endurance, coordination, and range of motion. Physiotherapy for bypass patients can include physical exercise, coughing, and deep breathing after surgery. Physiotherapists are also involved in patient education and planning a patient's recovery program once they return home.

Occupational Therapist

Someone who specializes in assisting people with disabilities to carry out daily living activities. These activities can range from swallowing, eating, and drinking, to getting dressed. Occupational therapists teach patients how to conserve energy during simple tasks, such as washing and getting out of bed.

Social Worker

Social workers help patients and their families deal with issues related to health and illness. These issues may include adjustment to hospitalization and dealing with long- and short-term effects of disease. Social workers also deal with financial or housing concerns and provide grief counseling. They help patients and their families plan for hospital discharge, which may include registering patients for rehabilitation programs, short-term respite facilities, retirement homes, nursing homes, or chronic care facilities.

Dietitian

The role of a dietitian is to identify how patients can improve their eating habits, to develop diet plans, and to collaborate with health-care teams to coordinate medical and nutritional needs. Dietitians also educate patients individually or in groups about high cholesterol, diabetes, weight reduction, and nutritional supplements.

Disclaimer: The above descriptions are intended as a general guide only. The roles of each type of staff member mentioned may differ slightly from hospital to hospital.

glossary

ACE inhibitor A drug used to treat hypertension and congestive heart failure, as well as to prevent heart attacks and worsening of angina.

Acute myocardial infarction A heart attack.

Allen's test A test performed on the blood vessels in the wrist to check if the radial artery can be used as a bypass graft. This involves blocking the radial artery in your wrist and checking that your fingers are still receiving blood via the ulnar artery.

Anesthetic A drug used to numb an area of skin ("local") or put someone to sleep ("general").

Analgesia Medications that are used to alleviate pain.

Anemia Not enough red blood cells. Red blood cells contain hemoglobin, the chemical that carries oxygen around the body. Anemia can occur after surgery due to excessive blood loss and is usually treated with a blood transfusion.

Anesthesiologist A physician who specializes in patient care during surgery, including pain relief, general anesthesia, and blood conservation.

Angina Chest pain caused by lack of oxygen to the heart muscle.

Angiogram *See* Angiography.

Angiography A procedure involving the injection of X-ray dye into a blood vessel and the photographing of that vessel on X-ray film. An angiogram is the still or video image produced by angiography.

Angioplasty An operation that widens narrowed blood vessels.

Anticoagulant A medication that "thins" the blood by blocking the activity of proteins involved in blood clotting.

Anti-platelet drug A medication that "thins" the blood by blocking the activity of small cell fragments in the blood called platelets.

Aorta The main blood vessel of the body, which carries oxygenated blood from the heart to the rest of the body.

Arterial graft A bypass graft for coronary artery bypass surgery that originates from an artery.

Arterial line A continuous-monitoring device that is placed in an artery, most commonly in the radial artery.

Artery A blood vessel that carries oxygen-rich blood from the heart to the body tissues.

Atherosclerosis A disease that commonly narrows or blocks arteries anywhere in the body. It involves the development of a fatty, calcium-rich deposit on the inner wall of the arteries called plaque that gradually builds up over many years.

Atrial fibrillation Quivering or rapid beating of the heart's two upper chambers.

Autologous blood donation Storing your own blood before surgery to be used after surgery in the event that you need a blood transfusion.

Autotransfusion Process in which a patient's own blood lost during surgery is returned to them afterward.

Beating-heart surgery Bypass surgery in which the heart is allowed to continue beating, thus avoiding the need for the heart-lung machine.

Beta-blocker A drug used to reduce blood pressure and/or prevent angina symptoms.

Blood banking *See* Autologous blood donation.

Blood conservation Techniques to reduce the amount of blood lost during surgery or reduce the chances of needing a donor blood transfusion afterward.

Blood count The number of blood cells in a standard amount of blood. Could refer to white or red blood cells, or to platelets.

Blood transfusion Giving blood to a patient through a vein to make up for blood lost during surgery. The blood can be their own or someone else's (donor blood).

Brachial artery The artery in the elbow.

Bypass surgery *See* Coronary artery bypass graft.

CABG *See* Coronary artery bypass graft.

Calcium channel blocker A drug used to reduce blood pressure and/or prevent angina symptoms.

Cardiac catheterization A procedure in which a long tube or catheter is inserted into the heart via an artery in the arm or groin. Cardiac catheterization allows physicians to carry out procedures on the heart, such as coronary angioplasty, without opening up the chest wall.

Cardiac enzymes Chemical markers in the blood stream that indicate the heart muscle has been damaged, e.g., by a heart attack.

Cardiac rehabilitation A support, exercise, and education program available to heart patients through their local hospital or doctor's office.

Cardiopulmonary bypass (CPB) machine *See* Heart-lung machine.

Catheter A narrow tube that is inserted into a part of the body.

Circumflex artery ("Circ") One of the three main blood vessels of the heart. It supplies oxygen to the muscle on the left side of the heart.

Clinical trial A test (of a drug or procedure) that involves patients.

Cognitive impairment Problems with memory or concentration. Can happen after bypass surgery, but is usually temporary.

Conduits The tubes used to bypass narrowed or blocked arteries during coronary bypass operations. *See also* Grafts.

Coronary arteries The arteries that supply blood to the muscle of the heart itself. There are three main coronary arteries, the right coronary artery and the two branches of the left coronary artery.

Coronary artery bypass graft (CABG) The correct medical term for "heart bypass surgery" or "bypass surgery." This surgery is carried out to relieve angina by creating a bypass around blocked or narrowed coronary arteries. The bypass itself is a short length of artery or vein taken from the leg or chest and grafted onto the heart above and below the blocked artery.

Coronary artery disease Any disease involving the coronary arteries. Most commonly used to describe blockage of the coronary arteries due to atherosclerosis.

Cross-matching A laboratory test used to find out which type of donated blood is suitable to give a specific person for a transfusion.

Dialysis The removal of toxic waste from the blood through an artificial membrane when the kidneys are unable to do so.

Double-vessel disease Heart disease involving two of the three main coronary arteries that supply the heart muscle.

ECG *See* Electrocardiogram.

Echocardiogram (Echo) An ultrasound image of the inside of the heart. Used to examine the size and function of heart structures, such as valves, and diagnose heart disorders. Usually performed by placing a transducer (probe) on the skin above the heart, and is painless.

Electrocardiogram (ECG) A recording of the electrical activity of the heart. This can be useful for diagnosing angina or a heart attack.

Electrocautery device A heated probe for sealing the cut edges of an incision to stop it bleeding.

Embolus A blood clot or piece of loose plaque that blocks a blood vessel.

Endothelium The normal lining of the inside of a blood vessel.

Erythropoietin A hormone that stimulates bone marrow to make more red blood cells.

Free graft A bypass graft that is removed entirely from its original position (e.g., a leg vein) before being grafted onto the heart. *See also* Pedicled graft.

General anesthetic A drug or combination of drugs used to put a patient to sleep.

Graft The tube used in bypass surgery to re-route blood around blood vessel narrowings or blockages. It is usually taken from a blood vessel in the leg or chest.

Heart attack The sudden blockage of one of the heart's blood vessels, resulting in the death of a portion of the heart muscle.

Heart bypass surgery *See* Coronary artery bypass graft.

Heart failure ("congestive" or "cardiac") The condition that results when the heart cannot, for one of a variety of reasons, pump enough blood.

Heart-lung machine Cardiopulmonary bypass (CPB) machine. A piece of equipment that temporarily takes over the pumping job of the heart when the heart is stopped during cardiac surgery.

Hypertension High blood pressure.

Hypothermia Low body temperature. Lowering the body's temperature during surgery decreases its need for oxygen.

Intensive Care Unit (ICU) A specialized ward that looks after severely ill patients or those who have had major operations.

Internal thoracic artery Also called the internal mammary artery. The artery that runs down the inside of the chest wall, which is used as a graft in bypass surgery.

Intravenous Through a vein, e.g., intravenous administration of fluids.

Ischemia Lack of oxygen to the tissues. If ischemia lasts too long it can damage the tissue or even cause the tissue to die.

Left anterior descending artery (LAD) One of the three main blood vessels of the heart. It supplies oxygen to the muscle at the front of the heart.

Left main coronary artery The most important blood vessel in the heart. It divides into the left anterior descending artery and the circumflex artery.

Left main disease Disease in the left main coronary artery. In severe cases bypass surgery is usually recommended, although angioplasty may sometimes be more appropriate.

Left ventricle The main pumping chamber of the heart.

Left ventricular function The pumping action of the lower chamber of the left side of the heart that circulates blood around the body.

Lipid-lowering therapy Medication to lower the levels of cholesterol and other fats in the blood.

Local anesthetic A drug that numbs the sensation of pain at the site of the injection.

Lumen The hollow space inside a blood vessel through which the blood flows.

Mammary artery *See* Internal thoracic artery.

Minimally invasive direct coronary artery bypass surgery (MIDCAB) Bypass surgery performed through small incisions between the ribs, with no heart-lung machine, instead of opening up the breastbone and stopping the heart as in traditional bypass surgery.

MIDCAB *See* Minimally invasive direct coronary artery bypass surgery

Myocardial infarction A heart attack.

Nitrate A drug used to relieve or prevent angina symptoms.

Nitroglycerin The most commonly used nitrate drug.

Non-invasive (test) A test not requiring any equipment to be inserted into the body.

Nuclear perfusion scan A test in which a radioactive drug is injected into the body to measure the flow of blood. This test is used to diagnose angina. It can be done in addition to, or before, an angiogram.

Occlusion A total (100 percent) blockage of a vessel.

Off-pump coronary artery bypass surgery (OPCAB) *See* Beating-heart surgery

OPCAB Off-pump coronary artery bypass surgery. *See also* Beating-heart surgery

Pacemaker The control center in the heart that determines how fast the heart beats. An artificial or temporary pacemaker is a wire that is inserted into the heart to control the heart rate.

Painless or "silent" ischemia Angina without symptoms of chest pain.

Palpitations A heartbeat that is unusually rapid, strong, or irregular enough to make a person aware of it.

Patency The length of time a bypass graft lasts without blocking up.

Pedicled graft A bypass graft that is sewn onto the heart at one end and remains attached to its original site at the other end. Usually refers to the internal thoracic artery in the chest wall. *See also* Free graft.

Percutaneous transluminal coronary angioplasty (PTCA) The correct medical name for angioplasty of the coronary arteries.

Pericardium The thin membrane that covers the heart.

Plaque The blockage responsible for narrowing blood vessels in atherosclerosis. A plaque is usually composed of tissue cells, fatty material, and, sometimes, calcium deposits. A complicated plaque is one that has become ulcerated (broken open), contains a blood clot, or is irregular in appearance. An uncomplicated plaque is usually a smooth narrowing in a blood vessel.

Platelets Small cell fragments in the blood that are essential for blood clotting.

Pleural effusion Fluid accumulation around the lungs.

Posterior interventricular or descending branch (PIV or PDA) One of the branches of the right coronary artery. It supplies blood to the inferior surface (bottom) of the heart.

Pre-admission clinic A hospital appointment for final tests and patient education several days or weeks before surgery.

Prognosis A prediction of the probable outcome of a disease and how likely recovery is.

Psychosis Strange behavior and loss of contact with reality, often with delusions and hallucinations. Can temporarily occur after bypass surgery.

PTCA *See* Percutaneous transluminal coronary angioplasty.

Pulse oximeter A device for measuring oxygen in the blood.

Radial artery One of the two arteries in the wrist that can be used as a bypass graft.

Renal failure When your kidneys do not work properly.

Re-stenosis Re-narrowing of a blood vessel that was once widened.

Revascularization The restoration of blood flow into the heart muscle by either angioplasty or bypass surgery.

Right coronary artery (RCA) One of the three main blood vessels of the heart. It supplies oxygen to the muscle on the right side and underside of the heart.

Saphenous vein A large vein in the leg that is used to bypass the blocked arteries in the heart.

Sedative A drug that lowers the level of consciousness and makes the person feel tired or sleepy.

Single-vessel disease Heart disease involving just one of the three main blood vessels supplying the heart muscle.

Stable angina Angina that is consistently brought on by exercise or stress and does not occur during rest or sleep.

Stenosis (plural: stenoses) A blockage or narrowing of an artery.

Stent A metal coil or tube used to keep a blood vessel fully open after angioplasty.

Sternum Breastbone.

Stool softener A medication that softens the bowel movements.

Stroke Damage to the brain caused by either bleeding from a burst blood vessel in the brain or blockage by a blood clot.

Suture A stitch.

Telemetry A method of monitoring the heart via electrodes placed on the chest.

Temporary pacemaker wire A metal wire that is inserted into the heart via the leg, arm, or shoulder, to temporarily take over from the heart's own pacemaker.

Thrombosis The process of blood clotting.

Thrombus (plural: thrombi) A blood clot that may block a blood vessel.

Transient ischaemic attack (TIA) A "mini-stroke" from which the person makes a full recovery.

Treadmill test A test for angina during which a patient walks on a treadmill with ECG wires attached to the chest, arms, and legs.

Triage A method for deciding who gets medical treatment first, according to the severity of symptoms.

Triple-vessel disease Heart disease involving all three of the main blood vessels supplying the heart muscle.

Troponin A heart muscle protein that can be measured in a blood sample after a heart attack or episode of severe angina.

Ultrasound An imaging technique that uses sound waves.

Unstable angina Angina that develops for the first time, suddenly becomes more severe, or occurs at rest.

Vein A blood vessel that carries oxygen-poor and carbon dioxide-rich blood back to the heart and lungs.

Venous (or vein) graft A bypass graft for coronary artery bypass surgery that originates from a vein.

resources

Heart Health Information

So You're Having Angioplasty... What Happens Next?
By Stephen Fort MD and Victoria Foulger RN.
SCRIPT Medical Press Inc.
ISBN 09688982-0-3

Mended Hearts Inc. (Canadian support available)
Support for heart disease patients.
http://www.mendedhearts.org

Heart and Stroke Foundation of Canada (Canadian)
222 Queen Street, Suite 1402
Ottawa, Ontario K1P 5V9
Tel: (613) 569-4361
Toll-free 1-888-HSF-INFO
(1-888-473-4636)
Links, news, and health tips.
www.heartandstroke.ca

Health Canada Heart Health Information (Canadian)
Links to heart health information.
http://www.hc-sc.gc.ca/english/azindex_ghi.htm#heart

Heart Information Network (U.S.)
Guides on heart attacks, hypertension, heart failure, arrhythmia, and stroke, plus news, nutritional help, and general heart health information.
http://www.heartinfo.com/

Heart Disease and Cardiology Information (U.S.)
News and information on surgeries, tests, risk factors, exercise, and heart-healing devices.
http://www.heartdisease.about.com/health/heartdisease/mbody.htm

Support for Bypass and Heart Disease Patients

Heart to Heart™ Program (Canadian)
1-888-473-4636
Sessions offered through the Heart and Stroke Foundation that educate patients and caregivers about healthy eating, reducing stress, and coping with heart disease.
http://www.heartandstroke.ca/
(click on "Heart Disease" and then "Support Resources")

The Zipper Club (U.S.)
Tel: 1-888-738-4220
or (509) 738-4014
Membership-fee site for survivors of open-heart surgery that includes a chat room, links, and merchandise.
http://www.thezipperclub.com/

The Mended Hearts Inc. (Canadian/U.S.)
7272 Greenville Avenue
Dallas, Texas 75231–4596
Tel: 1–800–AHAUSA1
(Ask for Mended Hearts)
Affiliated with the American Heart Association, volunteers who have dealt with heart disease are available to talk to heart-disease patients or their families about what they are going through. Site includes links, articles, and members bulletin board.
http://www.mendedhearts.org/

Stress and Relaxation Information

The Yoga Centre of Calgary (Canadian)
Yoga-related links.
http://www.yogacalgary.org/resources.html

The Transcendental Meditation Program (Canada/U.S.)
Find out the benefits of, and how and where to learn, transcendental meditation.
http://www.tm.org

Meditation Society of America (U.S.)
Concepts and techniques of meditation plus suggested reading.
http://www.meditationsociety.com

American Yoga Association (U.S.)
General information on yoga, how to get started and how to choose a qualified yoga instructor.
http://www.americanyogaassociation.org

Nutrition and Fitness Information

Canadian Wellness (Canadian)
A directory of fitness, diet, health, nutrition, and other wellness-related professionals and their services.
http://www.canadianwellness.com

Dietitians of Canada (Canadian)
Nutrition resources and news.
http://www.dietitians.ca

Dial-A-Dietitian (Canadian)
Tel: 1–800–667–3438
(Toll-free in BC only)
Tel: (604) 732–9191
Nutritional counseling, toll-free for British Columbia residents. Provides nutrition resources and links.
http://www.dialadietitian.org/

Health Canada's Nutrition Resources (Canadian)
How to choose food by reading labels, Canada's Food Guide, and research reports.
http://www.hc-sc.gc.ca/hppb/nutrition/index.html

Canada's Physical Activity Guide (Canadian)
Guide for how to get started on an exercise program.
http://www.hc-sc.gc.ca/hppb/paguide

Books

Adjey, David and Janice Holley. *Heart and Soul Cuisine: From the Estates of Sunnybrook.* Toronto: The Estates of Sunnybrook, 1997.

Cohan, Carol, June Pimm and James Jude. *Coping With Heart Surgery and Bypassing Depression : A Family's Guide to the Medical, Emotional, and Practical Issues.* Connecticut: Psychosocial Press, 1997.

Kessler, Seymour. *Heart Bypass: How to Prepare Your Mind, Your Emotions, and Yourself for a Successful Outcome.* New York: St. Martin's Press, 1995.

Levin, Rhoda. *Heartmates: A Survival Guide for the Cardiac Spouse.* Minerva Press, 1987.

Moosewood Collective. *Moosewood Restaurant Favorites.* New York: Clarkson Potter, 1996.

Stern, Bonnie. *Heart Smart Cooking for Family and Friends: Great Recipes, Menus and Ideas for Casual Entertaining.* Toronto: Random House Canada, 2000.

Wong, Stephen. *Heart Smart Chinese Cooking.* Vancouver: Douglas & McIntyre, 1997.

General Health Information

Telehealth Ontario
1–866–797–0000 (Canadian)
24 hours-a-day, 7 days-a-week hotline staffed by trained nurses with a least 5 years of experience. Direct links to 911 and emergency departments.

Canadian Centre for Activity and Aging (CCAA) (Canadian)
1490 Richmond Street
London, ON, N6G 2M3, Canada
Tel: (519) 661–1603
Fax: (519) 661–1612
Community information, events, research, and newsletters regarding aging.
http://www.uwo.ca/actage/index.htm

Canadian Health Network (Canadian)
General information about health for Canadians, including a section on heart health.
http://www.canadian-health-network.ca

Health Canada (Canadian)
News, disease information, and links.
http://www.hc-sc.gc.ca

HealthyWay (Canadian)
Health information from a Canadian perspective.
http://www.sympatico.ca/healthyway

HealthFinder (U.S.)
A service of the U.S. Department of Health and Human Services that connects you to publications, non-profit organizations, databases, Websites, and support groups.
http://www.healthfinder.gov

WebMD (U.S.)
Reliable health information including news, disease and drug information, health television guide, and tips for making a personal health plan and for searching the medical library.
http://www.webmd.com

Information on Alternative Therapies

The Canadian Naturopathic Association (Canadian)
1255 Sheppard Avenue East
North York, Ontario, M2K IE2
(416) 496–8633
Toll-free automated info line:
1–877–NAT–PATH (628–7284)
General information about naturopathic medicine.
http://www.naturopathicassoc.ca

Chinese Medicine and Acupuncture in Canada (Canadian)
Chinese medicine library, links, success stories, and practitioners.
www.medicinechinese.com

Ontario Herbalists Association
RR#1
Port Burwell, Ontario NOJ 1T0
(416) 536-1509
Toll free: 1-877-OHA-HERB
Learn about herbalism, find out how to participate in events, become a member, or use helpful links.
www.herbalists.on.ca

National Center for Complementary and Alternative Medicine (U.S.)
An official source of information, including links to other sites, current research, and scientific information.
Tel: (301) 231–7537, ext 5
Fax: (301) 495–4957
www.nccam.nih.gov

Alternative Medicine Digest (U.S.)
What's new in alternative medicine.
http://www.alternativemedicine.com

MEDLINE Plus (U.S.)
Information on herbal remedies.
http://www.nlm.nih.gov/medlineplus/herbalmedicine.html

Contact Information

Name of Current Family Doctor	Address	Phone	Fax	Email
Hospital	Address	Phone	Fax	Email
Name of Current Doctor (specialist)	Address	Phone	Fax	Email
Other useful contacts	Address	Phone	Fax	Email

Clinic Visits

Date	Time	Address	Doctor	Purpose

Test Results

Test	Date	Doctor	Purpose	Results

Current and Past Medications (including complementary therapies and supplements)

Drug Name	Date Began Drug	Purpose of Drug	Dosage	Side Effects	Dosage Instructions

Symptoms

Symptom	Date	Time	Cause	Severity on Scale of 1 to 10 (1=mild, 10=severe)	Duration

Taking Control of your Life

Rehabilitation Clinic/Other Wellness Center Contact Information

Address	Phone	Fax	Email

My Lifestyle Goals: Current Weight ___________

index

References to figures: *3fig*;
references to tables: *119t*;
references to More Detail boxes in bold: **4**;
references to Key Point boxes in bold italic: ***5***;
references to Self-Help boxes in italic: *12*

ACE inhibitors, 127, 130–131, *132t*
acupuncture, 115–116
acute normovolemic hemodilution, 35–36
alcohol, 88, 104
Allen's test, 58
anemia, 33, 34, 131
anesthesiologist, 38–39, 143
angina, 5–7, 9, 19, 20, **37**, *39*, 120
angiogenesis, 137
angiogram. *See* angiography.
angiography, 9, 10–14, *11fig*, *13fig*
angioplasty, 19, **25**, 14, 15–16, 20–24, **22**, **25**, **26**
angiotensin-II receptor antagonists (ARBs), 128
anti-arrhythmic drugs, 131, *133t*
antibiotics, 80, 128, *133t*
anticoagulants, 127, *132t*
anti-platelet drugs. *See* blood-thinning medications.
aortic bypass connector, 138
arterial grafts, 55–60, **56**, *57fig*, *59fig*
ASA (Aspirin), 9, 127
atherosclerosis, 2–3, 8, 9
atrial fibrillation, 81
autologous blood donation. *See* blood banking.
autotransfusion device, 72
beating-heart surgery, 24, 48, 66–70
beta-blockers, 126, *131t*
blood banking, 34–35. *See also* blood conservation strategies.
blood conservation strategies, 32, 34–36, 63
blood pressure, 106
blood-thinning medications, 72, 127, 129, *132t*
blood transfusions, 24, 32–36, ***35***, 72–73
breathing, 72, 74–75, 79
bypass surgery. *See* coronary artery bypass surgery.
calcium antagonists. *See* calcium channel blockers (CCBs).
calcium channel blockers (CCBs), 60, 127, *132t*
cardiac catheterization, 11–13, *11fig*
cardiac rehabilitation programs, 97, *108*, 122
cardiac risk factors, 4, ***5***, 8
cardioplegia, 62
cardiopulmonary bypass machine. *See* heart-lung machine.
cardiovascular disease. *See* coronary artery disease.
cardiovascular drugs, 125–128, 132, 133. *See also* coronary artery disease, medications for.
carotid endarterectomy, 26
chelation therapy, 117
chest pain, 5, 7, ***8***. *See also* angina; heart attack.
chest tubes, 75, 76
cholesterol, 106
clinical research trials, 136
cognitive deficits, 26–27, *75*, **82**, 83
complementary therapies, 114–117, **116**
consent, 31
coronary arteries, *6fig*, 11–13, *13fig*, 55–60, *57fig*, *59fig*, 62–63
coronary artery bypass grafts (CABG). *See* grafts.

coronary artery bypass graft surgery, 19, 48; advantages of, 20–22; as treatment for angina, 20; as treatment option for heart disease, 15–28, *17*; consent for, 31; future trends in, 135–138; history of, xi–xii; hospital admission for, 45–46; hospital checklist, *45*; medications for, 52–53, 78–79, 80, 94–95, *94*, 128–134; non-traditional, 65–70; pre-admission preparations for, 29–45; pre-surgery, 41–46, 49, 51–52; procedure, 47–64, **50**; questions to ask regarding, 29–30, *32*; recovery from, 71–117, 120–122, **121**; results of, 118–123, *119fig*, **121**; risks of, 23–27, **25**, 81–83, **82**; urgency of, **37**, *39*; vs. angioplasty, 20–26, **22**, **25**, **26**; vs. medications, 20, 21, **21**; work and, 36–37, 97–98
coronary artery disease, 1–9; diagnosis of, 9, 10–13, **12**, 14; lifestyle and, 99–112; medications for, 9, 17–18, 125–128, *132–133t*; risk factors for, 4, ***5***, 8; tests for, 9; treatment options for, 14–27, *17*, **21**, **22**
coronary endarterectomy, 62–63
coughing, *79*,
danger signs, ***8***, ***19***, **37**, *39*, *86*
decision-making, 15–27, *17*
deep vein thrombosis, 81
depression, 83, *96*,
diabetes, ***5***, 20, 21–22, **22**
diet, 88, 101–106, ***104***, *105*
digoxin, 130, *133t*
diuretics, 80, 128, 131, *133t*
doctor, when to call, ***8***, ***19***, **37**, *39*, *86*
donor blood transfusions, ***35***
double-vessel disease, **12**. *See also* coronary artery disease.
drinking. *See* alcohol; water balance.
driving, 87–88, *87*
drug therapy. *See* medications.
eating. *See* diet.
electron beam tomography (EBCT), 13
emotional changes, 95–96. *See also* depression.
erythropoeitin, 34
exercise. *See* physical activity.
follow-up visits, 86
free graft, 55–58
future trends, 135–138
gene therapy, 137
general anesthetic, 52–53, **53**, 129–130, *133t*
grafts, 19, 23, 48, 55–62, **56**, *57fig*, ***58***, *59fig*, *119fig*
heart, 1, 2, 54–55
heart attack, 7–8, ***8***, 82
heart disease. *See* coronary artery disease.
heart-lung machine, 23–24, 51, 61–62, *61fig*, 63–64
heart-protective medications, 130
heart rate, *92*
herbal medicines, 112–114, ***113***
holistic health care, 99–117
hospital admission, 45–46
hospital checklist, *45*
hospital staff, 139–144
impaired left ventrical function, **12**
incision care. *See* wound care.
intensive care unit, 71–76, **73**, *75*
internal thoracic arteries, 48, 56–58, **56**, *57fig*
laxatives, 131
left main disease, **12**, 16
leg vein. *See* saphenous vein.
lifestyle, 101–112, ***104***, *105*, *106*
lines and tubes, 52, 54, 72–73, **73**, 75–76, 81
lipid-lowering drugs, 9, 128, *132t*
magnetic resonance imaging (MRI), 13
massage, 116
medications, 124–134, *126*, *132–133t*, ***130***; after surgery, 60, 78–79, 80, 94–95, *94*, 130–131, ***130***; as

treatment option, 15–16, 20, **21**; before surgery, 128; during surgery, 52–53, 129–130; for angina; potential side effects of, ***111***, ***112***, *116*, *132–133t*, 134; pre-admission, **44**, 125–128. *See also* vitamins and supplements; herbal medications.
meditation, 115
memory problems. *See* cognitive deficits.
mineral supplements, 131, *133t*
minimally invasive heart surgery (MIDCAB), 48–49, 66, 68–70, **69**
myocardial infarction. *See* heart attack.
myocardial ischemia, 5. *See also* angina.
myocardium, 1, 2
narcotics. *See* pain management.
nitrates, 125, *132t*
nitroglycerin, 125
non-traditional bypass surgery, 65–70
occlusion, **12**
off-pump surgery (OPCAB), 48, 66–68
oxygen mask, *53*
pacemaker wires, **63**, 72, 76, 81
pain management, 78–79, 95, 130, *133t*
partial revascularization, 122
patency, 55
patient-controlled analgesia, 78–79, ***78***
pedicled graft, 56–58, *57fig*, 62
peer support, 96
pericardium, 2
physical activity, 81, 90–93, *91*, *92*, 107
plaque, 3–4, *3fig*, **12**
pre-admission procedures, 29–45
protamine, 129
quality of life after surgery, 120–122, **121**
questions to ask, 29–30, *32*
radial arteries, 48, **56**, 58–60, *59fig*
recovery, at home, 85–98; in the ICU, 71–76; long-term, 120–123, **121**; on the ward, 76–84; self-care and, 99–117, ***104***, *105*, *108*
relaxation, 114–115
results of bypass surgery, 118–123, *119fig*, **121**
risks of bypass surgery, 23–27, **25**, 81–83, **82**
robotic-assisted surgery, 137
saphenous vein, 48, 60–61
sedatives, 128
self-care, *17*, *39*, *86*, 87–117, *100*, ***104***, *105*, *108*
sexual activity, 89, *89*
silent ischemia, 6–7. *See also* angina.
single-vessel disease, **12**, 14. *See also* coronary artery disease.
sleeping, 87
smoking, 107
stenosis, **12**
stool softeners, 131, *133t*
stress management, 108–110, ***109***
survival rates, **21**, 123
tests, Allen's test, 58; for coronary artery disease, 9; post-surgery, 74–75, 77, 80; pre-admission, 38, 39, 40. *See also* angiography.
transmyocardial laser revascularization, 137–138
travel, 88
treatment options, for angina, 9, 16, 18, 20; for coronary artery disease, 14–27, *17*, **21**, **22**
triple bypass, 56
triple-vessel disease, **12**, 14. *See also* coronary artery disease.
urinary catheter, 75, 76, 80
unstable angina, 6
vein grafts, 55–56, **56**, ***58***, *59fig*
ventilator, 72, 74–75, 79
visualization, 115
vitamins and supplements, 110–114, ***111***, ***112***, 131, *133t*
ward, recovery in, 76–77
water balance, 80, 88
weight, 104–106
work, 36–37, 97–98
wound care, 80, 93–94